Traumatizing Linda:

Riding Cumulative Psychic Shocks into Dementia and Alzheimer's

By

William D. Dyer

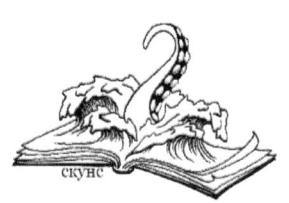

Copyright © 2024 William D. Dyer

Copyright © 2024 Salty Books Publishing, LLC

All rights reserved.

ISBN: 978-1964354019

Library of Congress Catalog Card Number: 2024918792

DEDICATION

I owe gratitude to some of the folks who were there when I needed them and continued to check in on me long after Linda—my wife, dearest friend, and loving combatant on the field of amatory battle, my marital partner for fifty-seven years, and my source of greatest support for longer even than that—succumbed to Alzheimer's: Frank Drollett, my oldest friend, fellow Corvette owner, and professional restorer of historic cemeteries who designed and set in place Linda's grave marker at the foot of my father's and mother's headstone; Melanie Payne and Mary Motter, Linda's oldest friends who've also had to deal with the loss of their spouses; Peggy Wallace, Linda's partner in teaching and fun at West Street School in Holyoke, Mass., who has also suffered the loss of her husband recently; Bobby and Irene Saunders who hardly missed a week in messaging cute cartooned uplifting blessings; Joy Sheets, our intrepid investment guru at RBC whose thoughtfulness included providing us with pizzas from Detroit, front row tickets to the RBC VIP tent in Blaine for a ton of food, drink, and a terrific pro golf tour event, admission at a fund-raiser for Minneapolis heavy hitters at which all we needed to do was eat wonderful food, bad golf for her and me, and always staying in close contact; Pat and Wayne Whalley, Linda's oldest and dearest college friends who entertained us by unfailingly beginning all of their letters with "How are you, we are all fine" and then following that up with a string of their most recent disasters; Michael MacBride, former student, dear friend, fellow writer, and technologist extraordinaire who has piloted my two books into print; and Heidi Thrall, whose professional care for Linda became an act of love.

I've saved my most effusive thanks to my little extended family for all they did for Linda and me: my son Chris, his wife Geana, and their four-year-old son Ronin of the star-crossed Cockayne's Syndrome who, destined to live a short life, lights up a room with his energy and enthusiasm—Linda got to know and love him before the worst of her illness visited her; Karen's two brilliant and unique kids Azra and Lee who looked after my Siamese cat Raj and helped me pick out another little one called Squeaky when I realized I needed more company; Karen's husband Hunter who made it a point to visit my flat after Linda died in between errands he ran on Saturday mornings, chat me up, and invite me over to enjoy examples of his and Karen's culinary delights.

But it's Karen who deserves so much more from me than I could ever repay. Always there for Linda. Unfailing in the support she continues to give to me. She managed and rode point on our last two moves; delivered groceries weekly to us during Covid; was always vigilant about researching Linda's psychic issues and diseases; took Linda to the hospital when I wasn't available to do it; made me laugh and buoyed my spirits when I'd mentally fallen down and didn't think I could get up; never shrank from getting into my face and tearing me a new one when I needed it most; wasn't shy about getting her hands dirty when I needed hands to help me do unmentionable things for her mom; was there for me shortly after her mom passed and helped me do the thankless yet deeply respectful job of helping me clean her up; and grieved hard and inconsolably with me, so much that I beat myself up over involving her too much in her mom's terrible end. She was my confidante. She saved me from myself. My heart is full to overflowing with what she has meant and continues to mean to me. I defy anyone to show me a daughter who encourages a father to travel for weeks with her to Russia, then France and Belgium, without serious disagreements and then to be planning to do it again in Chile and Terra del Fuego. There are no words.

And to you, Linda—you're still with me, now having returned, I persist in believing, to health and a happier self not far from me. Let me channel Brian Wilson and thoroughly mean it:

"God only knows what I'd be without you."

CHAPTER 1

"This is for all the lonely people..."
--America

What I've been trying to figure out as I've prepared the text that follows is whether there's a legitimate book to write and share with others here about my wife Linda, who died a little over two years ago. More to the point, should I write it? After all, although I'm a doctor, I'm not that kind of doctor. Where does a guy who's pursued a career in the humanities get off challenging diagnoses of what ultimately may have caused Linda's death? I don't question what other internists and specialists have told me about her long and deep depression, her dementia over at least thirty years, and the complications of Alzheimer's that ultimately suffocated her.

Beyond that, I'm deeply compromised and inculpated here in anything that follows; it's impossible for me to achieve total objectivity about her case because of our closeness over sixty-two years. For the last seven years of Linda's life, I insisted, against all reasonable arguments to the contrary, upon being Linda's primary caregiver even while admitting that I shouldn't have been.

In fact, it's possible to even label me as the antagonist of this piece. It's why I've been beating myself up for over two years now.

However, I've become more concerned about where Linda's Alzheimer's came from, and why. Are we dealing with an illness/career/degenerative disease that has its roots in chromosomal/genetic material? Does that mean, then, that this awful thing was inherited from one or both of Linda's parents? Certainly, Linda's mother suffered some considerable mental problems during her ninety-year life, evident in her decades-long depression and long bout with dementia. No way I can prove any of this--everyone's gone except Richard, Linda's four-years-younger brother, and his mental status is, at the very least, sketchy, with prolonged depression from a failed marriage and deflection and denial of his responsibility for any of it. He'd be no help. Besides, although he bore his sister no obvious animus, he refused to visit her during the last seven years of Linda's decline, even as I prodded him to contact her when it became obvious that Linda's death was nigh, and refused to acknowledge her death with a card or phone call. Said he couldn't travel. Back problems. I haven't heard a word from him since.

And at least a thirty-year bout with dementia might make it right for me to assume that Linda's mental health problems trailered off her mother's, to say nothing of the incredibly dysfunctional, nasty, and, during Linda's childhood, more than verbally abusive way her mother brought her up. Beyond those important markers, which might have cast the die for Linda's gradual mental decline, could one posit with some confidence that women are far more prone to developing dementia that progresses into Alzheimer's than men [1], a fact that may have further stacked the deck against Linda's mental health?

Although I don't have the data from Linda's health files to help me make a case (I'm not aware of any such files, though I've looked), I do have a long anecdotal history to draw from that

---

[1] See "Why Is Dementia Different for Women" in Alzheimer's Society (Mar 8, 2024) in https://www.alzheimers.org.uk/blog/wju-dementia-different-women# and many others.

speaks loudly, if not unequivocally, toward one. To bolster that case, I'm going to need to draw upon some support from a neurological expert who met a few times with Linda--initially, to elicit responses twice from her to a series of questions that would provide a gauge to evaluate her cognitive abilities, and, finally, to discuss the results of those tests with Linda, our (then) 44-year-old daughter Karen, and me.

In addition, I'm going to need to interweave in my narrative of Linda's story some important insights from the trailblazing book by child psychologist D.W. Winnicott (*Playing and Reality*), his former student Masud M. Khan's work in dream analysis and therapy (*Hidden Selves and The Privacy of the Self*), and, perhaps most crucially, Bessel van der Kolk's *The Body Keeps the Score: Brain, Mind, and Body in the Treatment of Trauma*.

But there's more. Let's, for the moment, call it collateral damage. It's likely that, during an average lifespan, a person is likely to be victimized by traumas of varying seriousness and intensity multiple times. All manner of shocks to our mental, emotional, and physical well-being assault us, ranging from childbirth, deaths, injuries from accidents that occur in the workplace or in the course of a normal day, the unanticipated end of relationships, the sudden intrusion of jarring news, a violent encounter, a betrayal, a crushing disappointment, panic attacks, a public embarrassment or humiliation, or failure to perform sexually. Those traumatic upheavals can occur because of something disturbing or violent that we have watched unfold or that has happened to us. Moreover, those incidents can be so traumatizing that our minds may be frozen by them, forcing us to replay them unbidden repeatedly and to be unable to let them go.

Linda had more than her fair share of such traumatic events. And I don't make that observation cavalierly. Some of them were hugely impactful. I'll later show that I, as Linda's lover, husband of nearly fifty-seven years, and primary caregiver in the last seven years of her life, was the author of a few events that contributed negatively to Linda's deepening and confounding traumatic bog that hastened her mental decline and ultimately led to her death. One of those was a major trauma that we shared and that she carried with her for decades.

In the following chapters, I'm going to embark on a discussion of each of these major traumas and how they may have impacted upon Linda's mental health and her relative vulnerability to dementia and Alzheimer's. I can't pretend to be speaking to a complete list of the traumatic events and experiences that Linda was subjected to during her life with me and before I showed up. That can't happen because my direct knowledge of Linda didn't begin until my nineteenth year when I met this sixteen-year-old beautiful young woman. Also, a definitive list would, I believe, expose me to some humiliation for some of the mistakes I made that contributed to what would become a life-long depression and adventure in anxiety. And, at least for now, I'm not concerned about the order in which I take up the individual traumatic events and the circumstances that surround them. I've opted to discuss them chronologically, although I could have presented them in the order of ascending importance for the developing state of Linda's mental health or taken them up "categorically," in terms of the relative type of trauma that impacted Linda.

But I'll begin with Linda's early years and the violent death of her father.

From all I've been able to gather from my direct interactions with her, my contemporary observations, and insights from others, Linda was a happy, out-going, exceptionally attractive, and active kid with a huge extended Italian family and a small circle of friends when she was able to stay around long enough to enjoy them. Her mom Dorothy Cassetina (Linda hated the name "Dorothy" that her mom chose for her middle name) married Orien Clark, whom she met in Washington D.C. during World War II while she was working in a secretarial position with the federal government. Orien had been active as a pilot during D-Day and afterwards flying DC-3s full of paratroopers to be dropped behind enemy lines as part of Eisenhower's big push preparatory to the beach landings at Normandy.

After the war, he moved with Dorothy to Rapid City, South Dakota, where his extended family was located, bought a tiny house on the outskirts of the city across the street from General Beedle School, worked in a radio and electronics store, celebrated the birth of a healthy baby Linda on July 16, 1946, and lived happily until he was called up once again to fly for the Air Force in 1952. Shortly thereafter, the then thirty-four year-old Orien was serving as co-pilot aboard an enormous ten-engine B-36 reconnaissance bomber that would crash into a foothill near the coast of Newfoundland during heavy fog and sleet in the early morning of March 18, 1953 [2], killing all twenty-three crew men aboard, including General Richard Ellsworth who led this covert training mission to test whether low flying techniques would enable the eleven bombers that followed his could enter American airspace unrecognized.

Lots of questions still surround this crash, the wreckage site of which has been preserved just as it was when the tragedy happened as a memorial to all who were lost. The mission, which included twelve B-36RBs and the full details of which were known only to Ellsworth, continues to be controversial. Because Ellsworth wasn't current on landings and take-offs with the huge plane, Linda's father, aided by co-pilot Pruett, took the craft into the air from the Canaries, and then Ellsworth assumed control along with Major Frank Wright.

Because the object of the mission was a test of whether the bombers could successfully over-fly the North Atlantic at extremely low levels (500-1000 feet) undetected, the plan was to operate with only radar altimeter and no radio contact until they reached Newfoundland, when map-based radar would be turned

---

[2] I'm indebted to a couple of sources for crucial details on Gen. Ellsworth and the crash. I'm indebted to a couple of sources for crucial details on Gen. Ellsworth and the crash. See https://www.baaa-acro.com/crash/crash-convair-rb-36h-25-cf-peacemaker-random-island-23-killed provided by the Bureau of Aircraft Accidents Archives as well as a more recent summary of the crash in https://rapidcityjournal.com/news/local/richard-e-ellsworth/article_a14bb162-6eb7-11e1-832b-001871e3ce6c.html

back on and altitude would be raised to clear the 900-foot coastal hills. Thus, navigation would be done solely by sextant and the stars until that point.

However, the weather quickly changed and worsened, the planes found themselves on the back end of a powerful wind shift that accelerated their progress toward Newfoundland, and, unbeknownst to the pilots, expected to hit landfall a good hour and a half before schedule and some 138 miles off course. This was soon to be catastrophic pilot error by whomever was actually at the controls of the plane—could it have been Ellsworth?—on which Linda's father was now a passenger. And, had it not been for a pilot taking a rest and peering down at the water only to see the tops of trees below him, the rest of that bomber squadron could have easily flown directly along the same low flight path to their mutual destruction. The grim huge debris field and the twisted wreckage left much as it was after it happened as a memorial tell it all—my daughter and her little family climbed carefully and respectfully over the site several years back--except the cost of those human losses to the loved ones left behind.

And that's where little six-year-old Linda enters the story. Unlike her two-year-old brother, suddenly aware of what she had lost but probably, like her mother, incapable of understanding the reality of it. It had been a non-combat training mission, and, after all, her dad had just recently been called back into service after having been mustered out at the end of World War II. She had deeply loved her dad; she related to me the thrill of accompanying him and her mom on hunting and fishing trips. And now, after the commemorations at the airbase, the renaming of it in honor of Ellsworth, and the somber burial at the National Cemetery at Spearfish which must have awed and stunned the little girl at the prospect of an endless sea of perfectly aligned grave markers (Linda and I were similarly awed by that scene when we delivered Dorothy's ashes to be interred next to Orien's, according to her wishes), there was only shock, loneliness, and grief for Linda. And she told me just how heavily and confusingly she remembered feeling it.

But that was just the beginning. Hardly any real time to grieve, and really no one to share that grief with. As soon as Dorothy had settled all the necessary paperwork as next of kin, disposed of Orien's personal effects beyond the ones that were highly portable, and sold the little house, she packed the two kids in the back seat of her '53 Pontiac, loaded up the trunk with their belongings and necessities, entrusted little Linda with the foldable national road map, and headed for California in the dead of night.

Note that this would be a perilous trip for a young mother under any circumstances a very long way from her Italian family roots in East Boston. But she was driving in the opposite direction! Eight siblings, she being the youngest in the pecking order among six older sisters, with a huge extended family of three hundred or so who were not nearly always mutually supportive of each other but who provided a protective umbrella against things threatening or unexpected. Instead of going home, Dorothy had been invited by a cousin to come to Cupertino, California, to live temporarily with one of her sisters while she determined what her next move would be.

But getting there would be an adventure. The commitment to and planning for Eisenhower's interstate highway system didn't get underway until 1956; that meant that cross-country travel was dangerous, incredibly time-consuming, and confusing. One major problem was a local and state spider web of mostly two-lane roads often ill-marked and in various states of repair. When Linda and I took our kids on our annual summer trips across the country and into Canada decades later, I always marveled at her seemingly innate sense of direction and her ability to map our progress. Linda told me all that navigational skill came from her being made the custodian of the maps in the back seat, calling out route numbers and connections to her mom as she drove and after they'd stopped along the road to sleep in the car.

In her grief, it seems that Dorothy didn't have a logical reason for taking that exhausting trip to the coast beyond the invitation. She was driven by pain and grief. And she and the kids wouldn't stay in Cupertino long. Soon Dorothy found herself loading the car once more for an even more challenging trip to seek the comfort and support of the Cassetina family in East Boston, and once again Linda was handed navigational duties. Kind of a harbinger of the out-sized responsibilities that her mother would thrust upon her in a few years in Massachusetts.

East Boston was mostly a happy landing place on Boardman Street in a very crowded three-decker apartment house just down the street from Star of the Sea Catholic Church and across the bay from Logan Airport. She had an instant crowd of friends in Dorothy's sisters' kids who either lived in the tenement or very close by. And there were the large family gatherings and wedding receptions that occurred, it seemed, nearly every weekend.

But Linda was far from fully adjusting to the loss of her dad. It'd be impossible to know if her experience in attempting to process Orien's violent death and her having been erratically shuffled from one coast to the other in such a short time brought on the fits of extreme anger that arose suddenly and that would become uncomfortably frequent in later years. Nonetheless, Linda favored me several times with a story of when she was playing with her cousins in the small, fenced back yard and how, after feeling abandoned by them, found a claw hammer in the near-by shed and threw it full-force through a screen door at a cousin standing on the other side of it. She didn't know why she'd done it, she told me, but was thankful no one had been hurt.

It would have been impossible to ignore Dorothy's passive and weak affect back then, which everyone who knew her would come to expect as normal: it's the operatic diva card she would continually play. What I'm referring to is grief taken to the level of theatricality. Whether due to the real grief of losing her husband so early in their marriage or a personality disorder, Dorothy was completely unable to initiate an action on her own. Whatever the reason for it, she projected helplessness and seemed to expect that everyone should actively volunteer to come to her aid.

It's an act that would get old fast but one that she never

tired of—the raised back of her hand held passively to her brow, her eyes closed, and whimpering, nearly a stereotype of the mourning Italian mother. And in her canvassing for sympathy, there was little room left for what Linda may have been struggling through. She did, though, provide then three-year-old Richard with affection and attention, as she would continue to do excessively over the next several years, to Linda's detriment and increasing emotional isolation. Richard became the object of Dorothy's attention almost as a fulfillment of another Italian cliché—he was his mother's son, and her only one.

It wouldn't be long before the little Clark family wore out its welcome in the increasingly crowded house on Boardman Street. Close quarters brought acrimony and argument, particularly because Dorothy wasn't contributing anything to the household finances, and the pressure to move out became overwhelming. It would be wrong to say that Dorothy initiated a search for a new house on her own. It's unlikely that she would have invested some of the money she received from Orien's insurance and Air Force death benefits into buying a house without pressure from her domineering sisters. And, when she purchased the new little house in a new subdivision off Granite Street in Braintree about forty-five minutes from her parents' house in East Boston (a house, by the way, which, uncannily, had been inspected by my father as a member of the town's planning board, with me in tow, before it was finished and found to be built from green wood), she did so because her oldest sister Francis, who lived directly across the street, instructed her to do so.

It was here that Linda's responsibilities in and around that house grew and a mother growing increasingly frustrated with her status as single parent and widow living on limited resources began to abuse Linda verbally and physically, constantly belittling her and punishing her physically for perceived shortcomings. All the while, Linda learned to make her own clothes with great skill and always had a part-time job throughout high school. Would that she had had the chance to share her grief, rage, and alienation with a professional who might have been able to help her process it. Instead, Linda carried the unexamined effects of her unresolved trauma with her into the next crucial stage in her development of a relationship with me.

CHAPTER 2:

"We can be heroes... just for one day..."
--David Bowie

Well...this is a tough one. It's tough because I was there, having inserted myself into Linda's life, muddling up an already damaged psyche and buried emotional life with my typically aggressive adolescent storming of her castle of virtue—or, at least, against an intrepid defense of it by Linda. A comic book version of *Romeo and Juliet* without the ladder and balcony (although I knew a very stupid and Shakespeare-stunted guy who tried that).

Please don't misunderstand—I loved Linda right from the start and to and beyond her dying day. It's just that my motives weren't entirely clear, at the very first sight of her and considerably later when I made some decisions with her tacit agreement—sexual and then marital--that were at first driven glandularly (of course—I was barely nineteen, nearly constantly tumescent, and in love) but then selfishly and callously. In the early portion of our growing relationship, I was unaware of the emotional and psychic traumatic incubus Linda was burdened with. All I really got to know was that Linda had lost a father, that she'd moved around a lot with her mom and brother because of that loss, that she'd had a normal dating history from the eighth grade on, and that she felt considerable animus toward her mother for restricting her freedom and imposing unreasonable Cinderella-like tasks upon her.

And, as we began to keep company, I could see what Linda saw in her mom. Lassitude. An existence of little activity, very late rising and then into a second bed made of the dilapidated couch in the small living room for more sleeping (sometimes never retiring to her bedroom at night) and interminable television-watching. When I first met Dorothy, I had already quit Tufts University amid my inability to cope with the death of my own mother the previous November, and, with the insistence that I get right back on the academic horse at Boston University, I was getting ready to do it again. My point is that I, too, was psychologically and emotionally damaged, with only one Holden Caulfield visit arranged by my father to a cliched shrink with pipe and arm patches on his coat to help me out of it. And, to make matters worse, I was totally alienated from my father, who was barely fifty, trying to manage his own grief, and meeting this rageful and rebellious nineteen-year-old essentially for the first time.

So, I wasn't really equipped, and far too self-absorbed, to evaluate the behavior of anyone else, but even I could see what was going on with Dorothy. TV on nearly all day and night. Refrigerator filled to the disgusting brim with indescribable and fragrant items that should have been thrown out long before. The absolute rarity of a properly prepared evening meal, and the impossibility of being able to clear a place on the cluttered small dining room table on which to eat it. I didn't really know what depression was then, but, if it had a name, its name was Dorothy.

But there was more, or less. Although she'd never gone to college (importantly, no one in Linda's huge extended family had until Linda broke that record), she had picked up a few things from the little reading she had done. She didn't know Italian, but she had picked up a handful of German expressions and immediately trotted them out to impress me. "Wie geht es dir?" "Was ist los?" That last one came out of her mouth a lot, with no realization by her of the irony implicit in it!

It took me no time at all—what a mental world-beater! — to understand, with Linda's respectful aid, that Dorothy was playing me, aware that my father was a "professional man," a civil engineer and a person heavily involved in the public business of Braintree. I more than suspect that she thought, incorrectly, that there was "money" and prestige in my background (and here I was, a little unkempt, long-haired "hoodsie" sitting before her), and she was encouraged to think that because my highly intelligent mom had drilled highly sophisticated vocabulary into my head by elementary school and how to use it—I was well-spoken when I was out of the influence of my scatological friends—I'd be quite a catch. She clung stubbornly to that illusion of my being high-born well beyond my brief and undistinguished cup of coffee at B.U.

But, just as importantly, she was self-absorbed. Her current straightened circumstances were other people's fault. She was still planning for her "main chance." That chance, she said, would be fulfilled by the successful completion of a real estate course that she and her best friend Rose had enrolled in and her intention to use it to become wealthy. But that would have required that she arise from Cleopatra's couch, get properly dressed, and get out there looking for an agency to attach herself to and some listings to show. Instead, she would talk for years about how her "main chance" had slipped away. There had been a new subdivision of summer cottages situated mid-Cape in the village of Popponesset and a particular property she'd visited that she'd set her hopes on. It was still affordable as nothing on the Cape is today, but, as was ever the case for Dorothy, she couldn't pull the trigger. As Linda and I would discover years later, she *had* the money, wherever it may have come from, but couldn't allow herself to part with it.

There was always something in her head that prevented her from committing her own money into anything involving risk. It wasn't that she didn't have the money. Linda and I pondered for years how she had been able to buy that house, live in it without ever working or earning a dime (we permitted ourselves some horrible speculations because she was an attractive woman!). She had several chances to marry again (there was the former boyfriend "Hoff" who in the late '70s convinced her to move into his impressive Albuquerque home with the promise of marriage. All she would have had to do was to pool her money with his demonstrably solid savings and pension from the Army Corps of Engineers, but she couldn't do it because that would have meant, to her, that she would have given up her own financial independence and her ability to leave all she had to her kids.

There were lots of men buzzing around that little honey factory. One of them, named Donald, came by at least once a week to mow the lawn and do house maintenance during which he would try to flex some discipline and authority over the way Dorothy was living; she strung him along for years. Another, a married telephone company worker named Robert, appeared at all hours. Many years younger than Dorothy, he carried on a very serious long-term relationship with her. In the end, she used Robert to establish long-distance phone connections so that we could talk to Dorothy wherever we might be. And there was another Bob who became her ignominious Cadillac chauffer (his car, of course) and personal whipping boy, cruelly mocking and humiliating him until he finally died of dementia, totally devoted to her to the end. She stole from all of them—from Bob even after he'd died--in small and large ways. And, yes, they were all married,

In short, Dorothy was a scheming, grasping, indolent piece of work who held Linda back at the same time as she was unforgivably permissive to Richard throughout his adolescence. This was our field of play as our relationship got under way.

And we went with it. When we first met in an open convertible on a cold mid-March night outside Boston Garden on the heels of an exciting Tech Tourney basketball game involving Braintree High, there was an immediate and electric connection. By Easter, we were dating, having lots of fun with our mutual friends, and conducting ourselves as a couple of teenagers in full amatory excitement. And there was no question that Linda was all-in; there was no hold-back in her open expression of how she felt about me and how she wanted the relationship to grow.

We attended her junior prom together and spent the summer in the glowing heat of our love. By the fall, we'd moved to the shore of the sexual Rubicon. Linda was holding on while holding very little back. At the same time, Linda and I were discussing what looked like a solid opportunity for her to become the first person in her family to attend college. Previously, she had underestimated her academic abilities, partly on the negative evaluation of her mother, but, after a long back-and-forth and weighing the very real and lesser opportunities she'd have after graduation, she applied and gained acceptance to Bridgewater State College and B.U. to become an elementary school teacher. It was a tremendous boost to her self-confidence, which would be nothing compared to what the public announcement at her graduation the following June of her having received a $4,000 per year military scholarship in the name of her father did to her sense of self-worth.

But that didn't change the increasing amount of skin we were showing each other. We knew where we were headed, but we were determined to put a hold on our relationship to see if going out with other people would cool things. From what she told me, she had a wonderful date with a student from B.U., and there was some kind of spark between them. But we were back together again, unable to keep our hands to ourselves, and, ultimately, that December, the drawbridge to Linda's castle swung open. We acknowledged to each other almost immediately after it happened that what we'd done wasn't a good thing.

And, within a month, we discovered why.

Suddenly, no job—I'd wrecked my car on an icy road, leaving me no way to get to my job. No money coming in. No prospects. No Merry Christmas. And then, at the very beginning of January, Linda's news that she had missed her period. We decided to keep her supposed condition to ourselves until time would confirm it, and it did. There's no way that I can put myself in Linda's psychic and emotional state. Of course, she was, as was I, terrified. I can remember as if it were yesterday my state of mind as I walked the mile and a half—I was car-less again—to Linda's house for the latest news. I was cravenly frightened about what was probably about to destroy our lives. No question in my mind that I'd stand with her come what may, but that didn't diminish my sense of twenty-year-old helplessness.

And then there was the beautiful and scared Linda. Guilt. The spectre of a brutally dark dead-end for her. In her mind, all that lay in front of her—graduation, perhaps a college education, the prospect of parties and proms that were about to unfold— was about to crash down upon her because she was being betrayed by her body, and me. There was the real chance that she wouldn't be able to finish high school, and the even worse probability that friends, fellow students, and family would never look at her the same way ever again. The laying-waste of reputation, which, back then, was the coin of the realm for a young woman. This was a heavy slam across the face for her, an assault upon who and what she believed she was. But, in my recollection, as deeply as she was fractured by this news, she kept her head up, didn't lose control, and, as we withheld her secret from her mom, she trusted that I would somehow come up with an answer.

Oh boy. Leave it to me! I still question whether she should have done that. A trip to her family physician in the company of me and her mother—no matter how humiliating—would have been the proper course, and, I might add in preparation for what was coming, the safe one. After all, this was about Linda, her health. But I was behaving and thinking like it was more than a little about me.

There's no way I can make myself look worse than to narrate my next move. A friend of mine, slightly older and shadier, had been in a similar situation with a woman he'd been dating. When I asked him how he'd handled it, he recommended a very questionable course of action. Once upon a time, he'd visited a man in a bar on Boston's Columbus Avenue for a bottle of ergot and quinine. He was told to have his girlfriend take it for three days and wait for a positive result. I asked him the unanswerable question about the safety of this mixture—I'm not sure if I really wanted to know—and then went to the library to try to research what he'd told me. Finding only some small anecdotal proof, I presented what my friend had told me (I absolutely hated having told someone else about Linda's situation) to Linda.

When she agreed to the plan, only, I'm sure, because she loved and trusted me not to do anything that might jeopardize her health and her ability to have healthy children in the future (how in the world would I have known anything about that!), I accompanied my friend Louie (yes, Louie) into the most crime-ridden and dangerous part of Boston—the "Combat Zone" at the nexus of Columbus and Mass Avenue—picked up and paid for the package at the tavern that was obviously a hang-out for whores and their pimps, and Linda began to take it immediately.

And to immediate effect. She felt a release of matter very shortly after the first dose. There was nothing to do then but for us to go to Linda's mother, lay it all out, and have the two of them repair quickly to their family physician. Dr. Sullivan's prognosis?—he said it was unclear whether Linda had ever actually been pregnant, and he pronounced the "medicine" that I'd caused Linda to take as no more than a harmless stimulant that sped up the expulsion of her menstrual material. She was fine, said the doctor, and would be fine in the future, at which point he prescribed birth control pills and sent her on her way. Throughout the ordeal, Linda said, Dorothy had remained mute.

I could never apologize enough for the nightmare I'd put her through, never mind exposing her to the ingestion of a substance of unknown quality or effectiveness dispensed in a bar room beneath the warren of whores' rooms in the heart of the

Combat Zone. Stupid, stupid, stupid. Dope slaps from all angles. The bitter end to any fanciful comparison between the naïve idealism of Romeo and Juliet and ours. I'd let her down. Put her at risk callously and needlessly. I've said before that stupid people are often the least likely to be harmed by their stupidity. It's the collateral damage—the innocent bystanders—that suffer.

A month after this incident, which says so much about the betrayal of my moral center, it was gone forever. Not a word. Over the next fifty-seven years of our lives together and right to the very last moment of Linda's life, we never once spoke of it.

But Linda's experience over those fraught two weeks left an invisible mark. How could it not? Tremendous anxiety. A threat to the very core of her being. An insight, I'm sure although she would never voice anything close to it, into who she'd come to know I was. It was a world-shaker, and, in some important ways, an accidental offer of a second chance for her to be something more than her mother had told her she was. A drawing-back from the brink and the opening-up of possibilities. But I'd keep on being her worst enemy, at the same time loving her beyond belief. If Linda's pseudo- or real pregnancy trauma shook her identity, that was nothing compared to the treat I had in store for her over a year later in the spring of 1965.

This was a relatively complex period for both of us, maybe more for me than for Linda at a time when I was attempting to get myself together somewhat responsibly, begin to find my feet in a more stable job with the hint of a future attached to it, and stop the chaos in my life. It was still very much all about me, my '54 Ford with Studebaker fins, and bad and alcohol-driven behavior with my friends. Priorities. I still remember stumbling drunk and shirtless five miles in a driving snowstorm with a friend into Braintree Square, stopped by two cops who made me walk a straight line before allowing me to wobble another three-quarters of a mile to my father's house to pass out for a few hours ahead of the court date I had in Quincy the next morning for I don't remember what.

But, I was starting to wake up. There'd be no more cups

of coffee at colleges; I'd burned those bridges. And after the patch work quilt of dead-end jobs—from short order cook at a GEM store; laborer for the local water department; office boy at my father's engineering firm in Boston; assembly line worker at a huge Coca Cola plant in Braintree; and jack-of-all-trades for Rocky Giancaterino doing sewer connections door-to-door—I'd gotten on to a more serious opportunity: working and training as an outside machinist at the old Fore River Shipyard in Quincy, now owned by Electric Boat/General Dynamics. From the first, I loved the work of wielding huge tools to strip and then re-install steering gear, pumps, and engines in the bowels of T-2 tankers being refitted as recovery ships for the space program. And, for the first time ever, I'd held a job for three straight months, giving me a chance to ponder a real future with Linda and to speculate with her when that might happen. After all, what could go wrong for a young woman deeply in love nearly mid-way through her senior year in high school?

From my construction and laboring days, I'd dreamt of owning a small fleet of ten-wheel dump trucks (it's crazy thinking about it now), shared my dream with Linda who was equally excited by my commitment to save fifty dollars a week to begin to make it happen. Wow. Castles in the air.

But it all fell apart at the Friday shift change a week before Christmas of 1964. Thousands of men were hurrying in different directions across the huge yard to punch out in the various tool sheds and machine shops and get on with their weekend. It was my bad fortune to literally collide with a man with head down rushing from the submarine basin. I recall saying, sincerely, "excuse me," receiving his "fuck you" retort, and, amongst those masses leaning in to watch, it was on. The fight lasted a mere ten minutes, with serious broken-bone facial injuries on both sides, and I wasn't fired immediately, but I would be a couple of weeks later for absenteeism in my attempt stupidly to file a Workmen's Comp claim.

What follows constitutes the single most significant threat to her fragile psychic and emotional well-being. It was the beginning of April now, a mere two years into our tumultuous relationship. I was working again, with no car, if "working" is sufficient to encapsulate the landscape work I was doing at various condo complexes in an adjoining town for minimum wage with the promise of learning the carpet installation trade and walking the three and a half miles home every day. Let me at it! But that was enough to jump-start my truck-owning dream again. And there was no turning back from pursuing our sexual relationship, particularly now that we had protection. But my guilt about what I'd put Linda through just before approaching the precipice of graduating safely from high school convinced me that I should make an honest woman of her. Of course. What a hero! Why not? What could go wrong? So much for the Romeo and Juliet parallel, except for the fatality that I hadn't reckoned with.

Hell, no one could say that I didn't mean well—could they? We were crazy in love, or, perhaps, just crazy. We were a Beach Boys song waiting to happen—"We could be married…and then we'd be happy…." And my plan for it all was insane. We'd drive to Concord, New Hampshire, in the morning, get the waiting period waived, do the blood tests, find a justice of the peace who would tie the knot, and be home in time for supper. In separate houses. My plan would require that we would need to live apart until I'd cobbled enough money for us to be able to find an apartment to move into.

Wow! Now that I'm a certified grown up and registered ancient person, it all seems so ridiculous. Somehow, Linda and I would get married, keep the secret from all concerned, and live separately. And that's exactly what transpired. In a moment of madness, Linda accepted my proposal, met me outside her house on the morning of April 23, Shakespeare's birthday, in the prettiest homemade black dress ever seen, and we drove at snail speed in my '54 Ford with Studebaker fins to New Hampshire's capitol, played gin rummy in the front seat while our blood tests were being processed, and stood before the honorable Marjorie Foote and a couple of office workers that she'd commandeered to be witnesses, and then drove home filled with the euphoria of what we'd just done. And then I dropped her off. "Good night, my baby. Sleep tight, my baby...."

And then, one month later and a little after two in the morning, she was suddenly awakened. Quite literally, by the pounding on the door of her mother's house by two Braintree policemen who were asking Dorothy if they could talk to the wife of William D. Dyer. "There's no Mrs. Dyer here," averred Dorothy. And then Linda entered and blurted out, "I'm Mrs. Dyer" (this would be the first time that she would have been addressed with her married name). "What's the matter?" That's what Emilia frantically asked when she interrupted Othello in the midst of throttling Desdemona.

What followed was shock and horror for her. The cops informed Linda that her secret husband of only a month had been in a terrible car accident involving a fatality, that his life was hanging by a twig at Quincy Hospital and that she needed to accompany them to the emergency room where he was being prepared for life- and leg-saving surgery.

I can remember Linda telling me about the catastrophic way that she'd been informed about what had happened to me, my problematic condition, and about the fate of the twenty-one-year-old driver who had been killed instantly after his car struck a tree at over 90 miles per hour. I can't be certain about when she told me all of it. I suspect that I wasn't conscious when she entered the emergency room, met my Aunt Ellen who lived very close by (my father was in Bermuda), and, sometime during the eight-hour surgery, responded together to the orthopedic surgeon who indicated that I'd flat-lined for a short space and that, given how badly my right femur had been shattered, he and his team recommended amputation. My little five-foot-two newly minted spouse wouldn't allow it, and, between Linda and Ellen, they fought for my leg. Some eight hours later, I entered Intensive Care with a full spiker cast with a board splaying and then yoking one leg to the other. But I still had my leg, thanks to the strong advocacy of Linda. And she was there in Intensive Care waiting for me, apparently composed and under control and dedicated to being with me for my recovery for as long as it might take. And, for a variety of reasons, that wouldn't be easy.

Trauma. Multiple traumas. It's still unfathomable to me as I'm narrating this stuff how she stood up to all of it. But, of course, as much of a shock as this legion of battering circumstances was to her—and I'm sure that she was for a part of the time fully involved in shock—she buried it, coming to my aid and supporting me. There's no question that this burial of so much of the psychic chaos she felt and would never really revisit at any time in the future with a professional therapist would cost her dearly.

But the pain of the double shock of her sudden public exposure from being married and then having to confront the very real possibility of losing a husband she'd yet to ever live with to a terrible car accident would soon be adumbrated, and through means she could never have guessed. Because I had no insurance, my father had an incredible mess to clean up when he quickly returned from Bermuda. There was the large financial burden of paying for what would be multiple operations to set the thirty-two broken shards around an eighteen-inch steel rod extending from the right hip socket to the knee. After a week in the ICU and another four ensconced in a bed at the end of a large ward, I needed to submit to another long operation to attempt a more stable re-setting of the leg, which resulted in success. The bills mounted up while at the same time dad was confronting my new wife for the very first time.

It's still hard for me to understand the machinations, first by Dorothy, then by dad, and then in collusion, while Linda was left out of almost all of it. It may have well been that Dorothy was experiencing her own state of shock, but I don't think so. She saw a practical way to cut her and Linda's losses by pitching, first to Linda and then directly to me as I lay helpless to deflect it, a kind of devil's bargain. Of course, Dorothy said, I understood how all of what had happened to Linda and to me had impacted upon her. She was only eighteen, after all, she said, still a mere girl, unable to properly address the college work that she'd probably be abandoning after a semester and a half. And, of course, she was merely a girl whom I had denied (there were lots of reasons why Dorothy knew better!) the natural and happy process of growing up, getting to know herself, and be with her friends.

But there was a way that I could immediately help in that regard. There was a dance that night, she said, at the Boston Army Base, and it would be wonderful if I'd give Linda permission to attend and enjoy herself. I was hurt and bewildered by her request. Was it total tone deafness I was hearing from her or something more pernicious? My bewilderment did not stem from any morphine-based meds I could have been taking. After my first night in the ICU when, under the influence of too much morphine after my first operation, I had experienced a fever dream of lying in the back of a pick-up truck and needing to swing my leg over the raised metal railing so that I could get out of it. As the foot of my injured leg had barely touched the floor, a nurse managed to summon help to get me back in bed, all the while screaming at me for what she believed was an intentional escape attempt. From that moment, I forbid the use of morphine-based drugs to manage my pain and have to this day.

No, I was completely aware and lucid as I listened to Dorothy, and I saw it for what it was—an attempt to withdraw Linda from interacting with me. I told her that she should pose the same question to Linda, and, when she arrived for a visit later, she told me that she had and that she'd been disgusted by it.

My father took a different tack. He bluntly posed the option of an annulment, trotting out the standard reasons for pursuing that path: it was quick, could be done within thirty days. Linda was so incredibly young, he reasoned. Her life would be ruined if she stayed with me, and she had a whole life in front of her. No reason, he said, to ruin her life as well as mine. Besides, what could she possibly do to help during the next seven months during which I'd be prostrate and helpless in bed?

On the face of it, hard to argue against what he'd said. If

I cared anything about her, which, I think, he had considerable doubts about, I'd let her go with no strings to live her life and forget these regrettable circumstances. This had been a game we'd been playing, he assumed, that could not stand when subjected to the current harsh realities. Never mind that there didn't appear to be any legitimate grounds for seeking annulment—he simply stood stubbornly behind the premise that we were irresponsible kids with no standing in the matter. And, contrary to his anti-Catholic and southern Mediterranean biases, he teamed with Dorothy in continuing that argument with Linda. She needed to be free to get on with her life; if she didn't, she'd bring all manner of regret, unhappiness, and shrunken dreams for the future by tying herself to an anchor.

But Linda refused to relent. She'd prove them both wrong, she said. And, when the ambulance left the hospital to deliver me to dad's house (largely because any other recuperative option would have been unthinkably expensive, and dad had had experience with round-the-clock home nurses during my mom's recent terminal cancer), dad viewed Linda as an inconvenient appurtenance. Excess baggage that must give way to the real caregivers.

That's not the way Linda saw it, though. She informed dad that she expected to be my primary caregiver and would take care of every medical and hygienic need without external aid. And she did, with growing competence, so much so that the voices of my father and Uncle John, who also lived with us, could be heard expressing surprise and wonder at how Linda was able to balance the part-time job she carried, full-time attendance at college, and her careful attention to my needs. It was tough work involving using the leverage of the spiker cast to flip me over regularly and keep me clean and free from bed sores.

I hesitate to say that she grew old fast under her responsibilities, showing unusual maturity under the strain of attending classes but doing no studying from the time of the accident to just before Christmas when the cast was sawed open and Linda and dad helped me downstairs to look at the tree. She'd barely passed all her courses, but she was deeply into academic probation. However, unlike me, she never quit. Years later when she applied to the University of Minnesota to pursue a Ph.D. in Curriculum and Instruction, she'd need to convince people that there were legitimate reasons for those bad grades as well as for the excellent academic record that she'd maintained in her two final undergraduate years. In another nine months, with her support, I convinced the Dean of Men at Bridgewater State College that I was worth one more chance, and he agreed to accept me if, should I need to be absent, I brought a note signed by Linda to verify my seriousness!

But Linda had to endure more unpleasantness while living in my father's house. Bigotry. Negative ethnic bias. I shudder to say that my dad expressed either of those toward Linda, but he surely did. I'd known since my childhood about my father's anti-Catholic bias. It had been expressed openly if not angrily. My sister Penny's best friend Marie lived at the top of the street, and every summer her father would take us to Nantasket Beach a couple of times each week. What a wonderful and generous man, but not to my father who grumblingly held his Catholic Irishness against him, and all Catholics. It was bad enough for Linda, in dad's eyes, that she was a Catholic, but even worse that she was Italian. Dark-skinned, oily, dirty, swarthy, uneducated immigrants who worked with their hands and too often operated outside of the law.

I don't know where any of this stuff came from, outside of the story that he often told me about the anarchists Sacco and Vanzetti who had held up a shoe factory in South Braintree in 1920 and killed the paymaster and his guard. Quite a celebrated and controversial trial leading to their execution, even though evidence of their innocence was suppressed. And dad grew up in South Braintree just across the street from the mansion of the Thayer family, one of whose highly prejudiced relations tried and found the pair guilty. Whatever the origin of his prejudice, he wore it like a badge; Linda and I often listened from our upstairs bedroom as dad and his brother regaled each other on Linda's ethnic and religious inferiority until I screamed for them to stop. They did, but their views about Linda's heritage, although unspoken from that point on, were crystal-clear. Linda suffered under that humiliation for the year and a half that we required to leave and rent a cheap apartment in an attic close to the Bridgewater campus. I know she felt it, and its effects on her were real.

CHAPTER 3

Life with Linda
As We Grew into an Interdependency

After we were able to escape from the hostile environment of dad's house, we were finally together, sharing the load. Living in dad's house had made a sensitive and highly emotional Linda cry frequently, and, notably, her mother never entered that house once while we were there—she was never invited. I'd been working a night watchman job at the old Hingham Shipyard. Stanley Carrabin, fellow gear head and donut shop denizen intentionally introduced me to the owners of their new marina start-up in March of 1966 to do roving patrol all night throughout the huge yard. I jumped at their offer—it was the only job that my slow-healing leg clad with a full leg brace could handle. It allowed me to get to my eight o'clock classes as well as a part-time gig pumping gas in West Bridgewater while Linda waitressed a couple of days a week at a classy restaurant in North Weymouth. We were honeymoon-happy to be on our own, and both of us began to excel in our studies.

But half-way through her senior year, during her teaching practicum at East Bridgewater Elementary School within walking distance from our attic apartment, I was about to pull her away from what had been a happy and successful experience. Faculty and students loved her there, she'd gotten wonderful reviews for her work, and they had signaled that all they'd need to employ her for the following fall would be a job application. We were happy paying $15 per week to live in our third-floor uninsulated crow's nest, and, given that Linda's job opportunity would provide stability and security, it looked like the ideal time for us to fulfill Linda's dream of starting a family.

But I had other ideas. Not content to finish two more years at Bridgewater, I began sending out applications to other universities in hopes of transferring into an economics program. On the recommendation of my sister and her husband who had graduated from New Mexico State University only forty-five miles from the Mexican border and had loved it there, I applied and was accepted for my junior year fall semester. So much for Linda's dreams. And so, uncomplainingly, with a fully-loaded several year-old car gifted to us in what seemed like a big kiss-off by my father's new spouse, Linda drove us away from everything that had become comfortable for her toward an uncertain next two years.

What we found when we arrived was a tiny cinder-block hovel in married student housing that allowed sand to pile up in the kitchen from under the door during Las Cruces' frequent spring windstorms, ant and roach infestations, and a high out-of-state tuition bill. We also had won what seemed like residence on the surface of the moon. Linda hated it, but, being the gamer that she was, she traveled some seventy miles west down interstate 70 to land a job at Deming Elementary school. The kids and administration loved her, too, but only for about two weeks when another job turned up for her in a Las Cruces third-grade class, and Deming's staff couldn't convince her to continue driving into a blinding morning sun any longer.

Nonetheless, as much as she loved her new job and it loved her, she frequently cried herself to sleep for the first eight months we were there. By happenstance on an early spring

Sunday at a miniature golf layout at the end of our first year, we became fast friends with a cluster of very happy and buoyant couples from New England which made all the difference for Linda's state of mind.

But I wasn't done yanking her around. I'd found a couple of unmatchable mentors at NMSU who convinced me to change my major from economics to English literature and I was off to the scholarly races. Of course, my commitment to an English major and History minor meant many hours away from Linda in solitude reading and writing. This would become a theme for me, a modus operandi in my several years of graduate school totally immersed in my studies and, as a consequence, neglecting the person whom I professed meant the most to me.

Because I'd performed so well in the program and garnered some key awards and recommendations, I began sending applications out to a number of prestigious Ph.D. programs, ultimately settling upon the University of Massachusetts at Amherst. Another wrenching, dislocating moving experience into uncertainty, guaranteed to send Linda visiting school department offices across western Massachusetts to find a position that would support my growing habit of seeking more degrees and committing most of my waking time away from Linda in getting them.

And, so, just when she had settled into another job where she was loved, appreciated, and fully competent, it was time to yank her across the country to UMASS-Amherst and another job for Linda. After an unpleasant and fractious summer living with Linda's mother and brother in their small house while we worked to gather enough money to pay UMASS's heavy out-of-state tuition, we found an excellent situation in the old mill city of Holyoke about a half hour from campus and within walking distance of the school where Linda would be teaching—Metcalf Elementary.

It was a huge, old rambling two-story house with a lovely little side porch and a big, covered second-floor porch in the front. We'd never had it so good! —the second floor all to ourselves, ten-foot ceilings, six enormous rooms, and an eat-in kitchen. Linda's trucking company-owning godfather (and I mean that label to include the underworld type) Bobby threw in a new electric stove and a leather Lazy Boy retractable that he claimed had "fallen off a truck." It was a wonderful three and a half years on that quiet street where we had two large litters of Siamese kittens, our first beautiful and healthy child Karen Colette after eight years of postponement, and found Norma, a woman two houses down who would be Linda's most important friend for the rest of her life and, when Linda gave birth in May of 1973, cared for Karen while Linda worked the remainder of the school year before taking maternity leave, which would begin at the start of the very end of the summer.

She had been over the moon with the anticipated arrival of Karen. She had blown up her petite little five-foot two-inch body into a beautiful, large, round, joyful exercise ball. I affectionately called her "the Little King." She had skied throughout the previous winter and had spent the spring crocheting little Afghans and knitting baby clothes. And Karen couldn't have been a more accommodating baby for a new mom. Linda had found her true role of being the mother that hers could have been but wasn't.

Meanwhile, we loved our landlords Chuck and Diane, who were barely older than us. Chuck, a lineman for the city electric company, was so happy that they'd found responsible renters that he found me a job on a road and sewer construction crew the following summer that allowed us to fund our long-delayed honeymoon to Bermuda, and, the following year, introduced me to the owner of a three-level bar in the flats of Holyoke where I got a job running liquor to all three floors. Linda was introduced to downhill skiing by Diane, and, for the first time in our relationship, I was watching her equip herself for a major physical activity that she enjoyed a couple of times a week.

But her joy was short-lived. Chuck and Diane approached us toward the end of 1973 with an opportunity. They had purchased a plot of land outside of Holyoke where Chuck intended to build their new house, and, before they put the two-story apartment building on the market, they offered it to us for $23,000 with no closing or realtor's fees attached. A bargain at twice the price even in those days before the fever of inflation hit the market. When I failed to convince my father to lend us the money—I understood that his doing so was a heavy lift only a few years after the medical expenses I'd put him through—we knew we'd be forced to move again.

That move proved a major disruption for Linda. The new very young landlord picked a fight with me over what he believed wrongly was a mess I'd created with some spilled refuse at the end of the driveway. The argument spread when he insisted upon inspecting our apartment at the very time when I and a few of my friends were moving the furniture out to be loaded into a truck. When I exploded and forced him out of the apartment because he was upsetting Linda and the baby, the argument only became more vigorous, with shouting and name-calling as we drove the truck up the street.

When we'd successfully moved all our belongings into the new apartment only a couple of miles away, I found Linda sitting listlessly on our couch with head bowed, completely silent, holding Karen close. She was unresponsive, and remained so for the rest of the evening until it was time to put Karen to bed. My first inclination was to label what I'd seen in Linda as postpartum depression, but that seemed wrong. Linda, as so many had observed, had loved being pregnant. It was something that she'd wanted and waited so long for. And she loved Karen ecstatically. Although I hadn't been allowed into the delivery room to support her, it was clear when I was invited in that Linda was beyond exuberant and bonding fully with Karen.

There had never been a minute, from Karen's birth on May 23rd and our hasty and nasty move at the end of August, of regret, frustration, anger, or disinterest toward Karen. Most notably, there were no observable mood swings in Linda's behavior. I had always affectionately called Linda my "sensitive plant" after a Shelley poem—that's because, when Linda was angry or upset or sad or heart-broken, she couldn't hide it. That emotion among the symphony of emotions that she normally displayed was inscribed on her face and all over her body. Although I've come to understand that postpartum depression can occur long after a mother gives birth, this was different. No rejection of her child. No panic attacks. No thoughts of hurting her baby. No. It took me a while to come to grips with it because this was an affect that Linda continued to display for a good part of the following year. It was depression.

Who knows how long Linda had been suffering from it? Was what I was seeing the emergence of the long-withheld and deeply buried feelings of worthlessness, abandonment, and rejection that she'd accumulated as a kid and left undealt-with, whether from her mother or me?

One thing was certain: we'd moved into an environment that cultivated that depression and caused it to grow. Jarvis Heights was a brand-new low-income apartment complex, and, when we moved in, it was far from completed. Construction trailers littered the site, building materials were scattered everywhere, and there was an air of danger about the place. During our stay there, we heard guns go off in apartments above and below us, and, once, when I returned from my liquor-running job after the bar closed at 1am, I drove into the parking lot to find several young men arguing and making a commotion. One of them was off-handedly brandishing a gun, not apparently to use but to show off. They met me as I exited my car and asked if I had a cigarette. When I offered them all around, they offered me a drink from their bottle of Southern Comfort. When I politely refused, claiming the late hour and my wife and baby upstairs as my excuse, we said goodnight, but I was on the alert from that point forward whenever I and my little family drove into that parking lot.

That winter I was hired on as a night watchman to walk hourly around the complex that included several empty buildings. On one frigid night, one of the construction trailers was broken into. I was confronted by the angry foreman of the project with news that a large roll of carpeting had been stolen during my watch and he was intent on blaming me for not standing watch with no break outside for the duration of my shift. I was later informed by the agency that hired me that the theft was an inside job timed to occur between the hours that I walked the area.

By the end of our stay at Jarvis Heights, because Linda was no longer collecting a paycheck, I was working three part-time jobs—in addition to the liquor-running gig and the third-shift watchman job that I'd continue to ride throughout my time in grad school, I held a teaching assistantship in UMASS's English Department that had me teaching two courses a year. Among the three of them, I grossed $7,200 for the year, just short of qualifying for food stamps, a reality that made our trips to the food store an abysmal experience. Anyone would have been depressed living in that environment, and, when, the opportunity occurred to abscond from that place at the end of our lease, we grabbed it.

Suddenly our fortunes changed from terrible to glorious. We had spent our spring weekends traveling from Amherst through Belchertown and South Hadley looking for a safe and affordable housing alternative. We found ourselves driving slowly down a quiet road just off a busy two-lane highway about a mile from the center of South Hadley and Mount Holyoke College that opened on a cul de sac bordered by twelve attractive brick apartment buildings, each containing two two-story apartments apiece. Most of the folks living there were older professional people who had resided there for years. We recognized immediately what a wonderfully humane living environment South Hadley was; our new residence would be considerably more expensive than what we'd been used to but beautiful and set on a little pond with large white ducks. Linda was happy again: lots of friends, plenty of bridge games with neighbors and cook-outs. But lots of in-built isolation for her while I continued to closet myself away from the family to study, write, correct papers, and prepare to teach—it took its toll.

And I'd be aggressively searching for a full-time teaching

job in just a couple of more years. But, before I go there, I can see a couple of critical themes developing here. First, as if I even needed to say it, there had been and were going to be many "moves" for Linda and me. And I'm certain that these moves took a greater toll on Linda than me. Why? —because Linda never complained about any of them and did them as more of a sacrifice for me, as a collaborative commitment to "take one for the team."

But there was always more in those moves for me than her. They were in aid of continuing my education or taking a job in line with my professional interests. All of them. And, reviewing the collection of them, I realize that they were far from necessary. Oh, sure, I got a lot intellectually and directionally out of the move to Las Cruces. I met Dr. Marion Hardman, one of the most important mentors I was ever going to have the honor of working with—the one who put me onto the idea that I could be a university professor someday and who insisted that I find a seat in a top-notch M.A./Ph.D. program. Who does that? Who becomes so enthusiastic about a student's ability and potential that she breaks a career-long rule of never recommending anyone for entry into a Ph.D. program before having completed an M.A. degree with distinction? Well, that would be my mentor Mrs. Hardman (although as entitled as any academic I've known to insist on "Dr.", she correctly never did) of the New Mexico State University English program. And I felt the pressure of needing to follow through on her evaluation of my abilities.

For a guy not as steady on his feet confidence-wise after the long recovery from the car accident, that was a head-turner. And her heart-felt discussion with me about my future preempted any other plans that Linda might have entertained. After having dropped out of two premier institutions, I was now on a run of four uninterrupted university years with the prospect of at least four more—and, as it turned out, it would be two years more than that because of my anxiety-driven penchant for over-preparation for the specific areas of literature that I'd ultimately be examined on and for the teaching I'd do in support of it. I was, as some might say, a "case."

So, in addition to the entirely unnecessary cross-country move to Las Cruces, there'd be the gigantic move from Las Cruces to the University of Massachusetts at Amherst. And, hell, I didn't need to act on the UMASS option immediately; I'd already been admitted without application to NMSU's M.A. program in English, which would have added stability to our lives for a couple of years, allowed me to kick the scholarly and pedagogical tires of a less stressful program where, as they used to say on "Cheers", everybody knew my name, and catapulted us out of married student housing into a more pleasant living arrangement.

But those weren't the only needless and stress-filled moves that I made Linda endure. Out of the ten moves we made during the first fourteen years (there were several more that I'll discuss later) of our marital adventure, six of them involved major interstate travel. Beyond the two I've mentioned, there were the moves directly related to my employment, although the second one would never have occurred if I hadn't opted to do the first one.

And that requires a little explanation. When Linda came to the end of her year-long maternity leave to nurture new-born Karen, she went back to work with a new assignment at Holyoke's West Street School to collaborate with a woman named Peg in a fully multilingual teaching venture. For the next three years, Linda loved Peg, the mostly Spanish-speaking kids, and the teaching environment unqualifiedly.

But, when she was about to reach her tenure year in Fall 1977 where absolutely nothing stood in the way of her continuing appointment (and, I must add, for her and for me real security such that we'd never experienced in our married life), I received the one positive response from the one hundred and twenty five letters of application for university jobs that I'd sent out. It was a terrible job market for anyone in the humanities that year, and it was getting late for English Departments to snag new hires—maybe mid-June. This one, at Indiana State University at

Evansville, wanted to interview me, they said. If all went well, they expected to hire me for the fall 1977 academic year. But, they warned, this would be a fixed-term position, with no possibility for conversion into a tenure-track job. The most that I could hope for, they said, was one or two one-year renewals while the person whose place I would be taking was making progress toward her Ph.D. coursework and dissertation. The salary? —a bottom-of-the-barrel $11,300. Yikes. A sum considerably less than what Linda would be making in a much more secure position.

I took the interview, which would have been paid for by Indiana State University-Evansville whether I accepted an offer or was rejected by them. And I was offered the job after an enjoyable interview except for some harshly worded questions about my long experience as a union guy and whether I'd stand with those who felt similarly should push come to shove (yikes again! —Indiana was and continues to be an anti-union "right to work" state, and union activity was strictly forbidden). But they were steadfast in discouraging me from thinking that there might be any life for me there at the end of my fixed term.

I told them that I'd need to talk to Linda about it, and we surely did. After lots of back-and-forth, I concluded that I should take it, that lots of my fellow Ph.D. candidates had repeatedly crashed and burned in their attempts to find a professional position, and several more had found themselves frozen in dead-end jobs like night auditor at the local Holiday Inn. Moreover, leaving UMASS's "Happy Valley" had proved impossible for some who chose to kick around town indefinitely rather than relocate.

Linda didn't really argue with me. She knew no one in Ph.D. programs across the country was getting employed. She understood that I was fortunate to get a positive response to one of my letters, never mind landing the thing. And imagine my amazement when the Humanities Program Director at ISUE stood up to introduce me at the fall university faculty and staff meeting and told everyone that over six hundred people had applied for the job I took! How hard-up were they! And what a crap shoot. Neither one of us was savvy enough to understand that I'd merely be cannon fodder until the person I was replacing returned. Nonetheless, Linda never expressed a doubt or reservation; it was all about and for me, she insisted, and fulfilling my professional mission.

But she had a lot more to lose than I did. A wonderful two-story living environment on a little lake replete with three years-worth of important friends who lived in the little complex and at the end of the road that opened out onto route 202 and quick access to Linda's job across the bridge into Holyoke. This may have been the happiest and most fulfilled that I'd seen her since our marriage. Intellectually, I knew all that, but, not feeling strong push-back (I never got that from Linda unless it was to protect me from myself for some bad social behavior), I called ISUE and accepted the job.

It was the wrong decision, flat-out. I think deep-down I knew it before I made it. I was playing this like it was the only job in the world, and maybe it was for that academic year. But we both could see that it was no trophy-winner. Basically, minimum wage. A blizzard of composition courses with a side order of World Literature to keep me interested. More than that, though, if both of us could have projected ahead to a few months of living in Evansville, Linda would have found herself without full-time employment, somewhat of a must due to my meager salary. Sure, she was able to put her name in for sub jobs—nothing in the world like getting a call at 6am and being told to drop everything she might have planned for that day and show up for sub work across town, probably with no lesson plan left for her to work with. And she would work them when they came available, but this would be tough duty for a mom with a six-year-old.

We talked about other options. Larry Haller, the husband of one of her very best friends several doors down who was a quality control manager for Sunoco Paper Products in Holyoke, had been covertly recruiting me for months during our evening bridge games and Saturday tennis matches. He literally laid his cards on the table one night when we were playing bridge, dropped a quality control handbook in my hands, and offered me a position for little more than ISUE had offered me. The job would require a relocation to upstate New York, and Linda delivered an emphatic "no" to the offer. I knew in my heart that I'd hate quality control, having applied very little of it in my own chaotic life.

But then there was the obvious. Turn my back on the job offer and keep applying. Hell, it was too late to catch on meaningfully that year, but so what? I had spent five days a week in a carrel in Mt. Holyoke's library drafting twenty-five productive pages of my dissertation for months, accumulating something close to 400 pages. Lots of revision required to bring the project home, and an analytical conclusion still to write. But, if I took the fall to sharpen and finish it, I'd be ready to begin the job application process, not AB.D. but with the dissertation in hand, defended, and the degree in my pocket at the turn of 1978. I'd be a much more attractive candidate. And, if all else failed, I could try to market myself as an adjunct to the many four-year and two-year colleges close by or move sideways away from teaching into a variety of other possibilities. A re-tooled job resume would show that I'd accrued lots of saleable skills. Nothing to lose. I'd logged a wonderfully satisfying year house-husbanding and bonding with Karen, and, with Linda returning to full-time teaching, I could help out by doing that again while finishing my degree and re-loading my job search.

That should have been our option. It was the healthiest one for Linda, the one that would have shown Linda that I was placing her first in our relationship after so many years of her putting me before everything. What wonderful morale and community at West Street School I'd had so many opportunities to see; the Friday afternoon volleyball games among faculty and beer parties were joyous even for non-joiners like me.

But it wasn't. I chose the apparently traditional path (Robert Frost would have mocked me savagely), accepted the job, and left Linda in the land of the might-have-beens. And what a regrettable move it was. As we always had, we U-Hauled the move, Linda driving the Pontiac while I dragged a tiny '72 two-cylinder Honda 600 behind the van. And off we went, leaving everything Linda cared about behind for a cloud of indefiniteness.

When we got to Evansville, we opted to purchase our first house. Given our finances, our choices boiled down to the tract house with the terrible kitchen and the non-descript straight ranch on a small triangular lot with a two-car garage converted into a large den with a huge raised stone fireplace. Unfortunately for us, the house was built on a flood plain, the slab that the garage had been built on wasn't raised when the den conversion was done, and you can anticipate the awful story I'll relate a bit later in this narrative.

And that's the one we bought. But, between the buying and the ultimate closing, we were living out of our small pop-up camper in Audubon State Park in Henderson, Kentucky, close to the race track on the other side of the Ohio River but a long commute to the university. For over two weeks, the contents of our moving van now in storage, I prepared for my professional days in a cinder block shower, donned my suit, and drove my little Honda 600 to campus while Linda languished in a campground filled with a bevy of bugs. Karen had a great time.

When we finally got our furniture out of storage and moved in, we came to realize that our neighbors to our right were very well-meaning and generous racists. Across the street resided the Luttrells, a born-again Christian family that seemed to have inside information on the Second Coming as well as the flood plain we were living on—if only we'd canvassed the neighborhood about our building's recent history. Dick and Phyllis, true to the evangelical thrust of their church, did their damnedest to convert us; Dick, in particular, showed up every evening after dinner with his tool box in his mission from God to volunteer for any project—and there were lots of them—we needed addressed. Good people, but with too much ulterior motive.

Additionally, once we moved into our little tract house which would, because of the location in which it was built, flood from extreme rains, run-off, and no storm drains, we would realize that there were no available teaching jobs for Linda. Yes, she did the sub work that was offered her, but most of her time was spent at home with Karen and a few close friends including the wife of my department chair that she was able to make. I don't know how I did it, but I finished the last chapter of my dissertation by late fall, hired a typist who needed all the help I could give in interpreting my eligible scrawl, and carried the four-hundred pages on the politics of use in the plays of Christopher Marlowe back to Amherst to successfully defend the thing by late spring of 1978. Small consolation for time it cost me with Linda and Karen.

It was that close friend, Joanne Gottcent, who did some extraordinary things for Linda and me. First, she had developed a great interest in women's health issues, specifically in preparing pregnant women and their spouses for a smooth and low-stress delivery. Linda and I enrolled in a series of her Lamaze classes. Besides being great fun, her classes taught us all how to breathe at various stages of the impending delivery, getting us to practice coaching the expectant mother to reduce stress, deal with pain, and, most importantly, focus. During the last months of 1978 until the end of April 1979, we practiced Joanne's techniques diligently until the time for Linda's final physical examination to occur at Evansville Hospital a week before she was scheduled to deliver.

And then the unthinkable happened. About eleven in the morning, I loaded Linda (Karen, fortunately, was in school) and the considerable precious load she was carrying into my old Pontiac LeMans (thank God I didn't choose to make the trip in my tiny Honda), and we drove across town toward the hospital. As I approached an intersection barely two blocks from the hospital showing a green light, I was struck on the left fender and door by a full-sized car driven by a young woman who had skipped school that day and had run the light without braking.

The violent impact drove our car up a telephone pole on the other side of the intersection.

Adrenalin kicked in. When the car settled against the pole, I found that Linda was conscious, lucid, visibly unhurt, but, as one might expect, in a full state of shock and anxiety. She was nine-months pregnant, for Christ's sake. I exited the car and moved to her door to see if I could help her get out; I even broke her passenger window, but the car was wedged against the pole. So, I did the only thing I could—I moved back into the driver's side, consoling and comforting her as much as I could while attempting to reassure her and me that she was alright.

But was she? And what about the status of the unborn boy she was carrying barely short of term? The paramedics arrived and, after firemen jacked open the driver's door, carefully removed her from the car and into the ambulance. And then it was the shortest of rides to the emergency room and a thorough examination that proved her to be uninjured physically and the baby safe.

Talk about trauma! And there were dangerous and difficult complications here. Linda wouldn't be coming home with me. Her obstetrician was fully aware that Linda had badly hurt her back the previous fall while helping me hang wallpaper. As soon as he and his team were able to stabilize Linda emotionally and address her back pain, her doctor indicated that she would be prepped for a delivery that could occur almost immediately. I was allowed to accompany her into the delivery room when her time came and to coach her in her breathing, which, given the back pain she was experiencing, helped her to relax and focus. The birth was normal although our new son Christopher was a large one, weighing in at nine pounds seven ounces, causing Linda plenty of discomfort.

But, as if that weren't enough, Linda was scheduled for a laminectomy as soon as her team of doctors thought it was safe. That meant some important collaboration between Joanne and me, first for me to take custody of Christopher from Linda after she had nursed him, deliver him to Joanne's house while I taught a class or two, go back to Joanne's again when it was time to feed Chris again and deliver him to Linda. Over the next several days, while she was being prepared for her operation and then going through her recovery, I repeated this process of taxi-ing Chris back and forth across the city to ensure that he got fed and bonded with his mom. Incredible. But it worked, thanks to the generosity and resourcefulness of Joanne. Through it all, Karen stayed during the day with the Luttrells, who lived directly across the street from our little floodplain.

Once Linda was able to come home, it took plenty of time for her to regain her strength and stability. It's fair to say that strength in her back never returned and that she was plagued with lower back pain from that point forward. Thankfully, a small army of women from our church and the neighborhood took turns delivering a myriad of hot dishes to the house. Tremendous, heart-warming, and unasked-for generosity. That was the first time we came to know what "hot dish" was.

I can't begin to gauge the effects of this trauma on Linda. She was probably inches away from being seriously injured, or worse. Not to mention Christopher! My recollection is that she didn't allow herself to dwell on how bad things could have been. Instead, she did what she always did—when she was able, she went back to being the queen of our little house, the loving mother of her two little kids, and an active participant in the business of her Anglican church..

But the positive effects of the back operation were only temporary and revealed a weakness in more than one of the discs in her lower back. That operation was the beginning of a series of back issues that, over the next thirty years, would cost her debilitating pain, another laminectomy and, finally, a spinal fusion that brought chronic pain, restricted movement, and, from that point on, a growing depression that would never leave her.

As I've noted, Evansville was a disaster for Linda all the way around. Two job renewals, each occurring at the last possible minute as fixed-term contracts in a right-to-work state, brought no psychological equilibrium for either of us. Nor did the social evening at our home we planned shortly after Linda was fully on her feet and could operate in our small kitchen provide any let-up in the upheavals Evansville delivered to us.

It's hard to pin down the exact date of that social catastrophe—I think it was in mid-June 1979 when I'd received formal notice that the person whom I'd replaced was dragging her feet toward her terminal degree at Indiana University and I'd been granted my last year-long extension. It was a particularly warm, still, clammy early evening that quickly turned into a heavy downpour. Being very close to the Ohio River, we were always worried about the possibility of floods, particularly because of our location in our little floodplain at the bottom of a steep hill falling off from a golf course located just above us. Our guests had arrived, we'd opened the wine, Linda began to cook, and, about an hour after the heavy rains had started, I walked out the kitchen screen door to our little concrete patio to survey the situation.

And then I saw it. A low wave of water descending across the yard behind us, through the chain-link fence and sweeping steadily over my little garden at the apex of our little triangular back yard. Everything started to move like a film in slow motion as the low wave of flood water progressed across the small backyard toward the house. Reacting in panic like a guy in a half-sunken rowboat attempting to shovel the water out of the boat with his cupped hands, I reached for a push broom leaning against the side of the house and, as the water reached the patio, began to try to push the water back furiously. Something out of a Far Side cartoon where a young man pushes a door in the wrong direction for entrance into the School for Geniuses.

By then, everyone inside had been alerted to what was about to unfold. As the rising water reached the double sliding glass door to the den, Linda, Karen, and our two friends madly moved bar chairs, couches, tables, and books—oh, the books!—to other areas of the house, and we all set about tearing the wall-to-wall carpet and its pad from its tack strips, pulling it as far into the center of the room as possible so that we could lift the fully-soaked and impossibly heavy rug onto chairs and stools as high off the floor as we could. Our efforts were made comically inadequate by the fact that the slider was set in its track at the exact height as the concrete patio, and the water simply rushed in.

Devastating. By the time the rain had stopped a couple of hours later and the water had begun to abate, we saw what we had won. Sheet rock surrounding the room that was soaked and discolored up to the three and a half-inch level, a great entrée for black mold.

Well, we got through it, but that flood was a harbinger of the second one we'd experience the following spring. Same result. Rinse and repeat, literally. Except that this time we were in the process of readying the house for sale! Yes, I was looking for a job again and doing interview trips from upstate New York to northwest Missouri to central Minnesota. After coming in second for a tenure-track Shakespeare position at the College of St. Benedict outside of St. Cloud, Minnesota, I was offered a one-year non-renewable World Literature job at the same place, and, without other options, I took it. But that meant uprooting my little family again, and, as much as Linda and I had come to loath Evansville and some of its attitudes—it had, after all, been the headquarters of the Ku Klux Klan at one time—despite the wonderful friends we'd made, this would be the toughest move for Linda.

How difficult it would prove to be began with the flood in May of 1980. Not as consequential as the first one, but catastrophic nonetheless because of its timing. Our little house wasn't much, but we'd put a bunch of money down on it that we couldn't afford to lose on resale. And that appeared to be what we were in for when the flood came, inundated the family room once again, and gave the already discolored and shriveled three and a half inches of white sheet rock another drenching. It was clear that we'd need to develop a radical solution—not just wholesale concealment of effects of the flood for prospective buyers but some major re-modeling of the back of the building most prone to water issues without breaking the bank.

With help from my neighbor Dick who had never given up on making us born-again, I gathered a small group of competent carpenters and concrete workers who worked for no more than the joy of helping us and solving our water abatement problems. Dick's next-door neighbor and his partner worked at the airport doing runway repairs. I'd done the same work for a short time a couple of years after Linda and I married and got our own place. Big jack hammers and concrete saws.

But Dick's neighbors had access to them and had a plan. If I could use the saw and jack hammer to cut through the four-inch patio slab and clear the rubble maybe a couple of feet away from the house, I could then dig down to the very base of the slab the house was built on and do some serious water-proofing, first with the appropriate tar and then the water-impermeable matted material to paste over it. After Dick's neighbors worked beside me to do the water-proofing on the back of the building and under the aluminum siding on the side of the house where the water had damaged the sheet rock, it was time for Dick to do what he did best—pull the sliding door out, open up the back wall fully to the elements, support the roof with two-by-sixes while his neighbor and business partner built a seven-foot form for a six-inch step into the family room on which the slider would now be set. All together, now—the Mickey Mouse Club theme song.

There really was no other feasible solution to our problem short of returning the family room to a garage or raising the entire slab of the great room to the level of the slab that the house had been built on. No way. This was as brilliant as it was cheap. We finished the job off with some angle-cut maple paneling to frame the door and some extra-wide new baseboard trim to conceal the damaged sheet rock. After we'd tacked down a new big rug remnant and sprayed a ton of room deodorizer, we cleaned up our mess, disposed of the refuse, and put the house on the market.

It sold in two days at a $12,000 profit. Yes, we left a bad

and leaky house to be repaired by an unsuspecting new pair of owners, but I felt no guilt other than what I'd put Linda through for the previous three years. Besides, we had a U-Haul truck to pack, a little Honda 600 to tow, and a car stuffed with two kids and our belongings and eight hundred miles to drive to St. Joseph, Minnesota, with no house to move into.

Dislocation upon dislocation. There'd been no time to look for houses to rent anywhere near the campus. In fact, St. Ben's was situated so far outside an urban area that renting an apartment was out of the question. It would have to be a house, and that would be expensive. Totally out in the boonies. Sprawlling farm acreage, and truly not the thing for Linda whom I'd yanked around from pillar to post and who desperately needed people around.

As it happened, we were able to contact a realtor who put us on to a large house unsold for over a year about ten miles from St. Ben's in a town called Avon. Shakespeare would have loved it. We got to know why this house was still on the market quickly. As I became fond of describing it, the house was perched on the median of busy interstate 94. It might as well have been, given that I had to wear earmuffs to deaden the road noise every time I went out to mow the back lawn. There was no playing in that big yard for the kids—too noisy. But across the street from us was Lake Woebegone, as Garrison Keillor had named it when he lived in this two-hundred-person town at the start of his career broadcasting from St. John's University just down the road.

It goes without saying that there was no employment available for Linda, meaningful or not, save for a three-month temporary federally assisted teaching job in the Albany Public Schools that she applied for in late winter. This was the gift-turned-joke that kept on giving for her since I'd made the decision to destabilize her life by committing us to anxiety in Evansville and then the inevitable extension of teaching positions of negligible worth to a one-year stint at St.Ben's before doing it all over again a year later one-hundred and twenty-five miles across the state in Mankato.

Nothing to see here in our quick and lonely stay in Avon. Just a blur of rides back and forth to St. Ben's to teach my classes, hold my office hours, try to do a little scholarly writing to make myself a more attractive job candidate, and get my next job search up and running. For many years, I've fancied myself as a modern-day Sisyphus, consigned by the gods to roll my damned rock up a hill and then to be run over by it going down, only to have to endlessly repeat the gratuitous process. What made it worse was that I'd enlisted Linda and the kids to participate in the rock-rolling.

It was clear now to me—I'm such a quick study in empathy and concerned observer of those I love!—that Linda was beginning to suffer, show psychological and emotional cracks around the edges. Little explosions of anger at the kids' occasionally cruel behavior toward each other. More frequent exasperation and loss of patience with the time I was taking preparing my classes and grading papers—even on car trips! Encroaching nervousness at the prospect of what could happen to us at the end of my contract and where we might go.

And, hell, even some of the nuns were asserting themselves on our behalf. They had gotten to know Linda and liked her, and they knew me either directly from social interactions or from hearing about my visitations to another sister's Spanish literature class to lecture and hold discussion on Cervantes' *Don Quixote*. Sisters Sheila and Linnea were particularly outspoken about trying to convince the administration to keep me on. Even long after we left, I'd encounter Sheila occasionally during some of my student trips to the Guthrie Theatre where she confided to me how much she wished we could have stayed.

But we were done, and we knew it. We said our final good-byes at a summer barbecue for English faculty at the lake home of the woman who had beaten me out for the permanent Shakespeare job. I had luxuriated months before over several students' review of her work in the classroom and how she had been the wrong choice (remember, Bill, that spite, according to

Dostoevsky's nameless narrator in *Notes from Underground*, is the smallest human emotion!).

Linda and I slipped away to find a couple of impossibly uncomfortable Adirondack chairs on the edge of the lake to discuss our problematic future. It was getting late. I still had unanswered applications out in the ether. There was still a chance. But it was nearing the end of July when even the infamous dead-ended one-year replacements were spoken for. For the first time in our marriage at this time of the year, we had nothing. What in the hell were we going to do? Where should we go if no jobs turned up? Holy apocalypse, Bat Man.

Counter-intuitively, I suggested Las Cruces. I reasoned, weakly, that perhaps some of the people I'd worked with at NMSU were still there and could put me on to at least part-time teaching. "Besides," I said, "we liked it there in our final year, had made good friends, and the climate was good. And maybe you could get another teaching job there." Linda immediately tossed my arguments to the curb—"it's been ten years, Billy. You know that your primary mentor Mrs. Hardman passed away, and chances are so have some of the other faculty you worked with. That, and all those friends are gone, scattered to the four winds, getting on with their professional and personal lives. I couldn't live there again."

Instead, she chose the Boston area and points north and west. "I've still got my Massachusetts teaching license. I accumulated eight years of full-time teaching, six of them at grade 5 in Holyoke. It's only been four years, and I had great recommendations. Some of our best friends are still there. And, if you couldn't get work teaching, there are all kinds of things you've done and could do."

Of course. I agreed totally. No one more pragmatic than Linda. And, if her plan sounds at all familiar, it's nearly identical to the one she'd spoken for and I rejected before we left for Evansville!

But, unfortunately or otherwise, it never came to that. The phone rang twice the following Wednesday—an embarrassment of riches--and on the other end of the first call was a voice emanating from Fort Kent, Maine. Yes, there really is an academic institution called the University of Maine at Fort Kent. A month earlier, I'd applied for a tenure track position there for a person to teach everything I'd ever dreamed of: renaissance literature, Shakespeare, Dickens. The thing virtually had my name on it. And I actually had relatives located pretty close to Fort Kent in Eastport, if any of them were still alive. Given the fact that my dad, located now in central New Hampshire, was sick with terminal cancer, this might have been my best chance to move close to him and help him if I could.

But, when I visited the campus which literally straddled the Canadian border, I had immediate reservations. I found that the student population numbered three hundred and fifty—six hundred if one counted part-timers. Only twenty-six faculty were employed by the college, which meant that nearly half the faculty had turned out for my interview. I couldn't imagine how I was going to be able to enroll enough students in renaissance and Dickens electives to make them "fill." And, although the little campus was pretty enough, there was barely any town. As for Linda's future employment there, the two biggest sources of employment—the SAC base at Loring and the potato industry— were suffering badly. With train service running only intermittently and annual snow falls predictably deep, I could foresee certain isolation for all of us, but particularly for Linda and her deepening depression. A meth lab waiting to happen. Even though the administration dangled $1,000 of moving money in front of me, the move, which would entail travelling over Lake Superior and across route1 through Canada, would be a huge undertaking. Linda was skeptical about my taking the position from the start, but, when the administration reneged on their salary offer to the tune of $2,000 because, as they put it, their original offer would have upset their salary structure, I pulled the plug.

But there was that second call, from Mankato State University. They needed to fill a fixed-term appointment for a

World Literature person who could teach lots of composition. The money wasn't terrible—actually, the same as the offer from Fort Kent before they rescinded it. Certainly, it was a one-year job—once more into the breach—with the chance of renewal for an additional two years. But, I rationalized with Linda, it was something, and, if offered, it would be a comparatively short move.

And so it came to pass that I showed up for the interview. A most strange one that occurred in a narrow conference room with ten faculty members, all accept one clearly at or past the end of their careers, seated before me at a long table. A long silence ensued among dour and undemonstrative people as if we were all attending a wake (perhaps we were), followed by several unchallenging questions that made me feel like little Pip awaiting an audience from Miss Havisham.

The kicker to the interview—there was no lunch—was a sit-down with the department chair, the dourest of all I had met that day who got right to the "wild card" of the job that I was about to be offered. I would be, she said, initiating a brand new T.A. program for the department to help draw numbers to a heretofore moribund M.A.-Literature program. It would be my job, she insisted, to recruit ten T.A.s (it was the end of July, for Christ's sake!), develop a course and training program to prepare these ten to teach Composition I, convene a two-week seminar in which we'd all develop syllabi, assignments, and grading criteria as well as supplementary readings for our courses, spend time evaluating real papers from previous courses I'd taught (why would I still have any of those? I threw away nothing!), and arrange to meet once each week with them to consider challenges they'd be faced with, along with a minimum of two visits to each T.A.'s class to evaluate their progress.

And now I knew why this job was still unfilled and why other faculty in the department hadn't jumped at the chance. For an untenured first-year person like me with no particular place to go if I lasted the year, this job amounted to professional suicide. True cannon fodder this time as if I was one of Falstaff's bankrupt recruits! If—and it was a long-shot, given how incompletely this major part of the job description had been assembled—I succeeded in building the program, with all of my still unknown T.A.s showing up and performing decently, after all of the evaluations of the participants, the program, and me had been weighed, with no students running to the dean claiming that the instructor of their Comp course was, in fact, no teacher and the course wasn't worth the cost that the student had paid for it, there was a chance I might be kept around for a while to do it all over again. But, if things went even slightly south (and I could see faculty from other departments crying foul about a union shop entrusting teaching jobs to non-teachers), I'd be history.

So where was Linda in all of this? I drove back to Avon and explained it all to her. She clearly saw the risks in accepting the job. But she wisely suggested that, should I succeed, whether I was kept on or not, I'd emerge with a set of skills that could serve me in a similar job down the road. Since the job would begin in a mere two weeks, we quickly loaded up another U-Haul, hooked up our collection of rust buckets—in addition to the big Olds Cutlass that I'd replaced the wrecked LeMans with and a vintage '64 Morris Mini Minor that was no bigger than the old Honda 600, along with a '72 Chevy Impala that Linda's mom had forced upon us while she was living with Hoff in Albuquerque—threw the two kids who had begun to take these moves as entertainment in Linda's car, and headed for Mankato.

But Linda had suffered from our initial move to central Minnesota a year earlier—I remember having to stop suddenly along with bluffs of Winona to let Linda out so that she could cry by the side of the road. She had begun to do a lot of that. Unaccountable crying and sitting by herself followed either by silence or no explanation. This had been a very strong and pragmatic woman for a very long time. She'd stood up to personal humiliation that I'd brought upon her, managed the kids and household finances, actively supported me through a period when I was attempting to get a medical explanation for my panic attacks (was I hypoglycemic? Was it diet? Now I understand what it was, and I'll address it later). Despite the back pain from her operation that she would never be rid of and plus what the lack of a permanent home had done to her, she had carried us all. Maybe Mankato would be that place.

But, if Mankato turned out well eventually for me, it wouldn't for Linda.

CHAPTER 4

Mankato—Not the Dark Side of the Moon, but Close

Mankato, a strange little city on the south side of the Minnesota River with North Mankato on the north side, known infamously for the largest mass hanging in the history of the United States—thirty-eight Dakota Indians. On the south side up on a high plateau sits the university. Almost immediately upon arriving in town, we looked for a lead on a place to rent while we checked in earnest for a house. We saw lots of bad possibilities, but were soon directed to a two-story modern apartment about two miles from campus overlooking a soybean field that might do the job temporarily.

Indeed, an apartment on the second floor was available, and, finding that no lease was required, we arranged to rent it monthly. That permitted us to drop our four cars and our pop-up camper in the large parking lot and to set about emptying the U-Haul. I remember it being hot, there being an uncommon number of other people on the second floor, some of whom lent us a hand, and far too little room inside to arrange and store our stuff.

Our immediate task was somewhat complicated—we needed to be able to live in this place as if it were our home while also using it as a storage unit filled with avenues of boxes filled with clothes, books, paintings, and personal items. More like a small warehouse than a living space. And no air conditioning. At night, Linda and the kids hung around in the halls while I sat on boxes and constructed my course syllabi. During the day, we raced around with real estate agents looking at very small houses that made us weep.

But finally we were directed to a place on the hilltop a mile from campus in a quiet little neighborhood that seemingly had everything we needed. 157 Meadow Lane. A Mr. Sjulstad was selling the house after having lived and brought up his kids in it for twenty years. And it was a young house, barely twenty-five years old. It had been built by two men who had taught in the construction management department at the university, and they had been ingenious in their use of space. The house was a split-level affair, with a powder room, kitchen, dining room, and living room on the first floor. Down eight steps were a large family room and a good-sized bedroom, with a fully finished basement another eight steps down, along with a large bathroom, primitive open shower, and a wealth of storage space. Eight steps up from the main floor were two bedrooms and a full bath.

But, in addition to the liberal use of oak trim on all baseboards and oak doors, the house was riddled with large hidden compartments for storage. There was one in our bedroom some five feet off the floor that we used to hide all our Christmas ornaments and presents we didn't want the kids to find (but they found them anyway). In Karen's room was a huge closet, enclosed in which was a very deep and wide rectangular space some six feet above the floor to store bedding. Our cats used it for sleeping, and, in fact, our kids made up beds and slept in it. There was only one garage, but it was enormous—at one time, I kept two full-sized cars and the Mini in there—and had even more storage space. The back yard was equally huge, with a beautiful Mountain Ash tree at one end and a mature Sunburst Locust located next to the large railing-ed deck. The yard was a privacy-seeker's dream come true, with a seven-foot hedge surrounding the back yard on all sides except for a little arbor-framed opening toward the back.

We were sold. Linda loved it, and I could see a brightening in her that signaled that she saw this as the home that, in large part, she'd never had. It was the biggest house on the street, and, because it may have been the only one on the street that had been sold more than once, the most expensive. But, at $65,000, it was a bargain in 1981. The country's economy was stuck in steep inflation. Interest rates were running as high as 20%, and we had no history with banks or home mortgages. Despite having to put down a huge down payment, we were looking at a blended interest rate of 12.5% for the first five years of the mortgage. Like most mortgages back then that weren't conventional assumable types, there was a five-year balloon attached to the loan which would require renegotiation of the mortgage when the balloon came due, after which we'd be required to re-mortgage at the going rate.

Of course, there was that crowded apartment that we'd been barely living and eating in, and we'd need to continue to do so for the next month until the official closing date. But, although I was inconvenienced by having to prepare my classes from what amounted to a storage locker, Linda was impatient but undaunted. She spent her time measuring up and buying material for the curtains she'd make for the entire house. Enthusiasm—I hadn't seen any in Linda for a long time, and I was thrilled by it.

But tough times of the usual sort followed for Linda once we'd settled in. It took a while to realize that Linda was not going to find a teaching job in Mankato. I can't explain why, but I'll offer a guess in a future chapter. As I've mentioned earlier, she'd logged lots of successful and praised full-time classroom experience. And she'd done a very creditable job as a sub over several years, always using her classroom time to advance the work that her students had been doing before she arrived and always leaving behind a careful record of the teaching plan that she'd enacted for the time she had spent so that the teacher she'd replaced could count on knowing where to pick up her own plans for her students. It seemed like a closed system, so strange for a university town where vagabonds like us were continually coming and going. She was well-known and respected, it seemed, for her short and long-term work—she was among the first to be called. Yet she was never able to break through and land a permanent job, and I know that puzzled and hurt her.

And then I got in her way again, big time. If I'd been paying strict attention to the rules governing various types of professional leaves, I could perhaps have averted doing so. But the first year in Mankato had become a difficult adjustment. I'd done well avoiding certain disaster running my new T.A. program—I'd had to step in to teach a T.A.'s class when he stopped showing up without telling me until I could find a replacement, as well as replacing another young woman who came aboard with no teaching experience and whose heart was pure but was simply emotionally unequipped to teach. But I'd had some difficulty adjusting to MSU's quarter system and the quick turnarounds in prep time to prepare each term's new classes. On top of that, we learned via a phone call that my dad had an incurable cancer that soon metastasized throughout his body and brain.

In April, my stepmother called to ask if I could fly to Florida to assist him in his flight back to their home in New Hampshire and then to the oncology unit at the Dartmouth College Hospital in Hanover, where he'd be given a last-ditch experimental chemo treatment directly to his brain. There was no expectation for him to live beyond another week or so.

Before I left, I explained the circumstances surrounding my need for a week-long leave, informing my department chair of my dad's dire prognosis. The form I was asked to file had no specific category for my reason for leaving, and, because the "bereavement" box seemed closest to what I believed I was claiming given my full expectation that my dad would be dead by the time I returned to campus, I checked that box believing that I had made an honest declaration, found a faculty member to cover my classes, and set forth on my sad mission.

I found dad in terrible shape, had to physically carry him on the plane, and got him home, where we found a ton of snow that needed to be shoveled so that we could transport him to the hospital in the evening. Dad was placed in an ICU with a chemo shunt in the top of his head, and we waited for the inevitable.

While he didn't die over the next several days, he was terribly weakened by the disease and the chemo, and the doctors humanely realized that nothing more could be done and sent him back home in an ambulance so that he could die peacefully in his bed. Although dad and I had butted heads over my misspent youth and my secret marriage to Linda for years, we spent a wonderful day and a half sharing stories about ourselves and reconciling. When I had to say good-bye to fly back to Mankato, I understood that I was seeing my father for the last time outside of a casket.

When I got off the shuttle in downtown Mankato from the Minneapolis airport, I found a phone booth and called home for Linda to pick me up. What I heard on the other end of the line was a tearful, terribly shaken woman. When I asked her what was wrong, she blurted out that my college dean had called her, angrily insisting on knowing where I had been and why I had spent eight days away from my job. Linda tried to explain that I'd taken my father to the hospital and then back home to New Hampshire to die. Dean Earley responded furiously, "Do you mean to say that Bill's father hadn't died during his time away from the university?"

Upon Linda's confused negative response, Dean Earley entered upon a rant: "Professor Dyer should have honestly stated his true reason for seeking a leave on the form he filled out. He misrepresented the reason for his absence, causing a number of people to be unnecessarily inconvenienced and taken advantage of while he was gone. This is a union issue that causes me to dock Professor Dyer three days without pay. When he returns home, inform him that he should call my office immediately." At that, she hung up, leaving Linda in shock.

I couldn't believe what I was hearing. Who does that (and

this won't be the last time I say that in this manuscript)! My initial response was shock followed by molten fury. What could have given my dean the audacity to explode all over my wife in the totally insensitive way she had? I asked Linda if she was calm enough to pick me up, asked for the dean's office number, and prepared to launch.

I know—literally, the dean was correct. I'd checked the wrong box on that faculty leave form inadvertently but with purity of heart. Another demerit for the Far Side genius. It was just like me not paying close enough attention to details such as this. But I knew something else, too. I was about to do something that could very well cost me my job and Linda any piece of mind she had left. And, typically, I didn't consider those implications over my white-hot anger.

I reached the dean. My congenial icebreaker was "how dare you address and upset my wife on the phone as you did? If you had a beef with me, I'd expect you to direct it toward me." To which she stated, "How could I? You were literally absent without leave. It's due to your own irresponsibility that I had to talk to her. You should understand that, if a parent dies, a faculty member must bring proof of that death via an obituary; otherwise, no reimbursement can be paid. In your case, there can be no reimbursement because there was no legitimate cause that you claimed. Therefore, I must penalize you with three days off without pay." My response? —"What an incredible lack of humanity and cruelty. You can go fuck yourself!"

As the bridge burned, I slammed the phone down on the hook, got into the waiting car, and told Linda what I'd done. Almost immediately, I knew two things when I said what I'd said to the dean: (1) I had said the thing that was true and wouldn't ever take it back; and (2) I might very well have to pay for what I said with more than three days' pay. Oh, sure, we couldn't afford to lose that amount of money in a bi-weekly paycheck with the mortgage payment looming. But I'd lit a match to the bridge Linda, the kids, and I were temporarily standing on. By rights, my pink slip might well be in my mailbox when I'd return to work after my suspension. More likely, what I'd told the dean could poison any chance for renewal for a second year that I'd be notified about within the next month. And, with crushing irony came the news of dad's death in just ten days, causing me to have to drop by the dean's office, revisit the 'bereavement" form for real this time, pay $3,200 for last-minute tickets for all of us to attend the funeral and wake just outside of Boston, and return three days later with the obit and the receipts.

And did Dean Earley hold what I said against me? No. Not only did she renew me for another year, but one year after my third one-year leave, she knocked and entered my office and happily told me that, because of all the good work that I'd done in the interim, she'd converted my position to tenure track and applied the three years I'd already put in toward my eventual tenure. Remarkably, although I retained my skepticism about the often arbitrary and capricious decisions this four-foot nine bowling ball of a martinet made, I understood that almost everything she did was for the good of the department and college. When the time came to choose a new Humanities director, Dean Earley recommended me for the job. For the remainder of my career at MSU, she remained one of my biggest supporters and I one of her most important allies and advisers.

But all of that doesn't erase the mark it left on Linda's fragile psyche. Whereas I rode the exhilaration of the renewal reprieve into the first five weeks of summer school teaching, Linda did what she had always done in the face of a crisis—she chose not to talk about it. Lots of personal catastrophes over the years blanketed with silence. It's not that we didn't talk and laugh and share the things that meant so much to us daily—the kids, our friends, the passionate love we felt for each other. Linda had always been incredibly demonstrative and open sexually with me, and I felt no diminishment in my physical attraction to her. Quite to the contrary. The kids were adjusting to a real home, and Linda would soon find friends for life at Mankato's Anglican church. And, while at the hospital a few years later while getting a hysterectomy, she met another preparing to give birth—more on that later.

But her old habit of hiding her disappointments exacted a price. Having always battled a weight problem, Linda saw her weight suddenly balloon, whether due to the hysterectomy or not. But the frequent wild mood swings that she began to experience most likely were dividends of that operation (and it was a tough one, given the fibroids her body had developed), and she acknowledged as much. Soon, she plunged into menopause, and she took the changes that overcame her badly. Extreme and frequent hot flashes plagued her, fouled her moods, and intensified her depression.

I remember that, in 1988, without any notice, she announced that she had begun to see a female psychologist, and, from all appearances, those visits improved her sense of well-being. She clearly felt an empathy from that professional, but the relationship was short-lived. In less than a year, her weekly visits stopped when her psychologist took another job and moved away. When the relationship ended, it was like Linda had lost a close friend and confidante. Although I urged her to look for another therapist, she refused, almost as if this particular woman was irreplaceable.

But even with as much emotional pain as she was feeling, Linda never quit trying to find a place for herself in Mankato's teaching community. In fact, when she couldn't win a position in the Mankato Public Schools, she took another tack. MSU's Education Department had just constructed an M.S. degree in technology; Linda applied and gained entrance. Within a year, she'd finished her course work and written her thesis that resulted from her research into distance TV systems and their practical implementation that that prepared her to create such a set-up for enabling MSU professors to teach interactively to sites all around southwestern Minnesota.

Having received the very first M.S.-Tech degree from the program in 1987, Linda applied for several jobs at area public schools looking for a Technology Director. She interviewed well, but failed to land one, placing second three times to male applicants. Visibly undeterred, she applied for a one-year opening in MSU's Curriculum and Instruction department to supervise student teachers across southern Minnesota. Right up her alley, it seemed. She succeeded in being awarded one of two available positions, and she was finally happy to be doing what she believed she should have been doing all along.

But things were about to go south in a big way for her, and I bear some responsibility for what would happen over the next few years. She was as happy as I'd seen her in years. She was gainfully employed. People across the Education Department had come to know her well as a student as well as a colleague now, and she felt valued and appreciated. She loved the work which took her into many different school systems from the Twin Cities to across the southwestern prairie, but her job was ending soon, and she was confronted with an important decision. Women in the department wanted her to become a permanent member of the faculty, but that would require getting a terminal degree. A huge and daunting commitment for someone in her early forties now, and there were absolutely no guarantees of her being able to finish a Ph.D. or to roll it into a full-time college teaching job.

We talked plenty about it. Gaining acceptance into UMINN's Ph.D. program was no sure thing. Given her terrible grades at the beginning of her undergraduate experience, she faced an uphill battle. She'd need to excel at the analogy test which was an approved option to the GRE exam. And it was unclear whether her age would prove a detriment to her application.

But there were other more consequential considerations. She'd need to commit to what I'd had to commit to—serious time away from the family both while studying at home and at the U's library. Hell, the U's campus was eighty miles away! And Linda would need to travel back and forth to the U to take her courses as well as find a way to enroll in a full load of course work during the summer. That clearly meant time away from the kids while entrusting me with the job of caring for and feeding my twelve-year-old son. Big competing forces pulling at her. Guilt. Anxiety. Plus, there was the real question of whether, at forty-three, she wanted to work as hard as she'd need to. Did she want it badly enough to make these sacrifices?

Of course, we talked vigorously and anxiously about it. I knew she could do it, told her so, and promised to support her in every way to make it happen. At the same time, we were getting advice from friends working in academia whose advice Linda valued who attempted to discourage her from pursuing a Ph.D. There was nothing personal in their negative advice. In one case, a friend who had some special insight into the profession warned Linda against it. "Older applicants at this moment are not valued as much as they should be," he said. "Besides, overall, there are too many terminal degree-holders out there who haven't yet found jobs. The more degrees you accumulate, the more likely you are to price yourself out of the hiring process. I doubt very seriously that you'll find gainful employment with a Ph.D."

Much of what he counselled was true. A lot of grunt work required for very few college and university teaching positions. It would be crazy to recommend such a path for someone in mid-life just for the sake of holding an advanced degree. What a worthless trophy! And I'd begun to counsel my own grad students in English away from applying for entrance into Ph.D. programs for the same reasons. "Only if you've really distinguished yourselves, can't live without doing it, and have a clear idea of the areas you'd be pursuing," I'd been warning them.

So why the hell wasn't I issuing the same prescription to Linda? After we'd discussed as many pluses and minuses to doing a Ph.D. as we could think of, I gave her the tacit go-ahead. I told her I had confidence in her abilities, academic and pragmatic—she'd proven as much in completing the difficult and hands-on work she'd done for the M.S.-Tech degree. I saw the confidence she'd gained from evaluating her student teachers. And I told her that I felt strongly that the ground was shifting employment-wise for late-forties Ph.D. candidates, especially women. Of course, even if I'd been loudly talking through my worn Red Sox hat, she'd have had her head turned by me anyway. Hell, I cared about her, right? I'd never steer her wrong.

But I believe now that I did. I meant all the things that I told her (what a damned unrepentant know-it-all I am!). I believed that she'd find a university job at the end of the rainbow. And she did. As it turned out, there were plenty of jobs for people of a certain age with the proper credentials just like her. But I couldn't shut off that nagging voice in the back of my head that kept telling me that I might well have had a more complex agenda. Oh, wouldn't it be wonderful if she was able to find a job at a four-year school! Who knows—maybe I could apply for a job where she was working and work alongside her! Perhaps we could team up on the presentation of conference papers and writing projects! And wouldn't our prospects for retirement be gangbusters if the both of us were putting money away for that rainy day!

Bullshit! There's a fly in the ointment, as my mom used to say. Something rotten in the state of Minnesota, thought my inner-Hamlet. How much of what I was advising Linda to do was about her or me? And we're not just talking about any prospective Ph.D. student. We're talking about Linda of the deepening depression; Linda of the wild and crazy consequences accruing from hysterectomy and menopause; Linda of the fragile ego who had been fighting for some recognition and acceptance; Linda, the good and devoted mother who understood her kids had reached an age when they'd need her more than they knew. A true generator of guilt there. Yes, I knew all that, and I'll say again that I loved Linda like nobody's business, but that I gave her the thumbs-up just the same. Wow.

Starting in the fall of 1989, she had begun her adventure at the U. Lots of stress. Just what the doctor ordered (which doctor? —me? Perhaps I'd forgotten that I'm not that kind of doctor and cannot write prescriptions). No problems with her application. She had aced the analogy test, all her recommendations were superlative, and her grades in the last two and a half undergraduate years and her work on her M.S. degree were exemplary. And she continued to do great work, to intersect with the two Johnson brothers, experts in collaborative learning, early on and develop the essence of a focus for her dissertation—a collaborative learning study involving fifth-graders, social studies, and technology.

By the beginning of summer 1991, Linda had finished all her course work except for three courses that she'd need to complete in residence at the U. That was the hardest part of the journey for her. On Friday evenings, she'd leave us to drive to the west bank of the university and check in to her dorm, where'd she'd stay until Sunday afternoon before traveling home. There had been more than just a little pressure on her since she'd begun her program; she'd had to spend large blocks of time away from us, and the guilt she'd felt for being an absent mother had grown. There were exams to take and consults with her dissertation advisors, the Johnson brothers, for determining a clear direction for her research study and a specific classroom in Mankato to set it in motion. But, by mid-July, she'd finished her residence and returned home, quite certain that her good friend who she'd met in the hospital after her hysterectomy would make room for her and her study in her fifth-grade class in Mankato.

But there were two things yet that she was driven to accomplish. Her weight had gotten out of hand since she'd begun her Ph.D. work. She'd heard from her physician when she went in for a check-up that he was starting a weight loss program that would be open to the community. I attended the first public meeting of the group with Linda, and I became skeptical when the doctor explained that the program would focus on fasting. That would mean a largely liquid diet and multi-vitamins supplemented with lots of rice cakes. I couldn't imagine anyone not nauseated by the prospect of a steady diet of rice cakes—barely any taste to them at all with the texture of Styrofoam insulation.

But Linda was as driven ("driven" had become a behavior pattern for her) to do the program as completing her Ph.D. course work, and, within about eight months, she'd lost between seventy-five and eighty pounds. Not only that, but she began to power walk with a couple of women at the church, so fast that I couldn't keep up. She and I both knew that she'd lost too much weight—perhaps twenty-five to thirty pounds more than she should have. She looked gaunt and angular, but she protested that she felt great about herself and was filled with energy.

A pattern was emerging here. Depression to exhilaration and back again. And soon she began complaining about gut and kidney pain, leading her back to the diet doctor's office and a diagnosis of kidney stones. Sounds just a little like malpractice. I don't know anyone else in the program who had to endure having their kidney stones blasted by ultrasound so that she could pass the residue, but she did. That was the end of the diet, although she continued with the rice cakes because she'd come to really like them, and, by the time Karen began her sophomore year at Bryn Mawr outside Philadelphia, she'd gained back those twenty-five pounds, leaving her looking like a beauty queen, as good as she'd ever looked since our marriage.

Which left her with the last item on her to-do list: to visit Karen at college and spend several days having fun with her and her roommates. What came out of that trip was not only a physically beautiful, healthy, confident, and self-assured woman now comfortable in her own skin and accomplished, but a person who'd fully bonded with her daughter, been on her own without my interference in social situations in which other men found her as attractive as I did, and was ready to return to finish her degree.

And she did. Through the rest of the fall of 1992, she entered her friend Mary's classroom, conducted her study—"An Investigation of the Effects of Cooperative Learning on Computer-Monitored Problem Solving"—involving three fifth grade classes and their teachers, analyzed her conclusions, and, in late spring of 1993, defended it at the U. And, in early June, she walked across the stage, with her bemused mother in the audience (she was well along in her own bout with dementia), and proudly received her degree.

In the glow of that magnificent personal achievement (it

mattered very little that her mom was too far gone to appreciate its significance), Linda could have no idea about the humiliations that lay just ahead for her. To set the stage, I must flash back to 1987 and the end of her year chasing around student teachers at MSU. It had gone well, she thought. No glimmerings of failure or disappointment or ill-feeling about it. Her friends in the department congratulated her on a job well done and wished her well. And, at the end of that year, at a departmental end-of-the-year party, Professor Lydecker, her advisor, thanked her and commended her on her work. She even had Linda and I over to her home in St. Peter for dinner the following week.

So, at some point in the next two years, Linda asked her if she would feel comfortable writing on her behalf for acceptance into the U's doctoral program. She did, Linda gained acceptance on the strength of her application package, and, somewhere in the last few months of her doctoral research study, Linda came to Professor Lydecker again to ask her to update her letter in anticipation of applying for full-time faculty openings. Again, she consented unreservedly.

What followed in the summer of 1993 is still hard for me to think about. There was no shortage of available tenure track openings for a person like Linda with her proven skill set, teaching experience, and Ph.D. in hand. Just about every job that Linda applied for extended her a campus visit and interview. Although most of these openings were at Catholic schools with no teacher union and smaller starting salaries, Linda didn't care. She merely wanted, after so many years of waiting her turn, to return to a full-time permanent classroom and do what she knew how to do.

So, when Linda came in second at the first job she interviewed for at the College of St. Thomas, she didn't think anything of it. However, when, during the next week while interviewing at St. Mary's University in Winona, something shocking happened. The interview had gone exceedingly well; Linda had performed a science teaching lesson that left everyone impressed. But just before she said good-bye to the department chair, he took her aside and said, "We loved your presentation and the skills you've shown. I'm sure that, under other circumstances, we'd hire you on the spot. However—and I have to think that you're unaware of this—there's a very negative letter in your file. What's even worse, it was written by Professor Lydecker at MSU, your teaching supervisor. Everything else in your dossier is solid and positive. However, this one letter—I'm going to advise you to pull it from your file immediately after having read it carefully and replace it with another positive one. I'm so sorry. I wish things were different. I sincerely wish you success in your job search."

Oh, my. Like a shovel to the face. Linda staggered out to her car, somehow managed to drive herself the three and a half hours to get safely home, and then collapsed in a heap.

Let's think about this for more than just a minute, shall we? One walks through not one but two comprehensive processes, blithely and confidently stands for questions about her competence and readiness to do the job she's there to interview for, gives a public presentation to both faculty members and other interested parties, and discusses her future with administrative officials including the university president while thinking she knows all there is to know about herself and her credentials when, in fact, she doesn't. Now that is a humiliation. Not just a little like interacting an entire day with other professionals while unaware, because no one has informed her, that she's operating with a compromising dress malfunction, but worse.

Hard to describe the range of emotions Linda displayed when she rushed into the kitchen as I was preparing supper. I believe I said something impossibly insensitive like "How'd it go?" without looking up from the stove. She'd been crying. Her body was visibly shaking. Her state of confusion and betrayal were tattooed all over her, even before I expressed my concern and asked what had gone wrong. But she was about to explode in anger.

I couldn't believe what she told me. I held her as she

reiterated her embarrassment in excruciating detail, and I felt my face flush with embarrassment. How does someone recover from an event like this? How does one prepare oneself for the next interview at a different university, not knowing whether someone who had known Lydecker and had caught a whiff of her appraisal of Linda might surface?

And, once again, who does that after writing a solid letter but following it up with a bad one?

For the rest of the night, I did my best to console Linda, but she had been physically and emotionally wounded and was unappeasable. We'd head to the university early in the morning, I promised, access her dossier and pull the letter. But what then? There was no way to phone Lydecker—she'd moved on to an administrative post at—consider the irony!—Bridgewater State in Massachusetts, now a university. But there were the contents of the letter to read. It's gone now—Linda destroyed it once she had fully digested its contents. And it was as bad as the department head at St. Mary's said it was. I can remember only one declarative sentence from that page-long letter: "Do not hire this person." No other letter in Linda's file remotely like this one. Only Lydecker's.

It's not too much to label this as a traumatic/traumatizing event. Good God, it was ruinous. And Linda, still stunned by the letter's rejection of her competence, had no clue where it had come from. Yes, she'd interacted with Lydecker on a regular basis, during bi-weekly seminars with the supervisors in her charge as well as in the normal interactions that faculty members customarily have with each other in the halls and at meetings. But she could recall nothing in formal and informal interactions that might have spurred such animus, such a confident dismissal of Linda's abilities or conduct. Nothing.

I'm going to interpose my own experience in this attempt to understand what had gone wrong here. And I shared all of it with Linda at the time. As a full professor for thirty-three years at MSU and more years elsewhere, and as a many-year veteran of university-wide committees charged with evaluating faculty applications for promotion and tenure as well as chair of my own department's personnel committee, I'd come to know that one of my most important professional responsibilities was to write letters for students and faculty, to be a referee in the purest sense of the word. If a student came to me with a request for a letter of recommendation for a job, acceptance into a grad school, or a scholarship, I understood the gravity of what I was about to commit myself to do.

That's why I approached the task with each student with complete candor. If, in my experience with that student, I felt unable to write a positive letter, I was duty-bound to tell that student so, and then, in response to the obvious concerns that such a student would express, specifically why I couldn't. I owed it to that student to tell the truth and itemize it. It would then be up to the student to either accept the letter containing all the dings and scratches or gratefully move on to another referee who could write a positive one.

Furthermore, for me there was nothing more important in my interactions with students than those letters. My name would be on them, and, thus, my reputation. And, knowing how crucial to their personal and professional advancement these letters could be, I always offered students the opportunity—before I sealed and sent them to their files—to read them. If I'd misrepresented anything in my comments about their work or abilities, I wanted them to be able to respond. No surprises. No personal scores to settle. That's because my assumption was that, on the official form students provided me to type my evaluations of their work and their prospects for success, there was always a box at the top of the form to check that indicated that my letters of recommendation would be kept confidential from them.

Seems simple, doesn't it? But, then, what the hell had been the meaning of what Professor Lydecker had done in Linda's case? I can't get inside her mind, nor am I certain that I'm equipped with all the facts in the case. But, on the face of it, she wrote her letter with malice a-forethought. She had reached an inner understanding that Linda shouldn't be teaching, even after having written an effusive letter of support for her entrance into a doctoral program, the outcome of which would be a teaching job. Lydecker seemed to be asserting that Linda had accumulated all of her prior experience as a teacher under false pretenses or incompetent vigilance by those she had previously worked for, and should never be entrusted with training others to teach when she wasn't a good teacher herself. Lydecker was also a teacher with many years of experience, and she had written, I suspect, many other such letters for students in the past. And, hell, she may have even been right in her assessment of Linda and her work, although neither I nor Linda have been able to gather any direct evidence of that. A little more on this later in the book.

But, if Lydecker had felt as strongly as she had shown so clearly in her letter, and if her first concern as the supervisor of those out in the field observing and advising future teachers should have been to weed out those who might do damage to both individual future teachers and the reputation of the department, why the fuck didn't she speak directly and privately with Linda about her concerns when Linda was employed by her to evaluate student teachers, about what others might have told her about Linda's work, and attempt to coach her into behaviors and strategies that would, in her mind, improve the quality of her work and personal interactions?

That wouldn't mean that, when push eventually came to shove, she couldn't still write her letter for Linda in ways she really felt, but any such letter probably would have been considerably more nuanced, indicate Linda's growth as a reflection of Lydecker's positive mentoring, and be available for Lydecker to share it with Linda before she sent it off to Linda's file. I don't mean to be indelicate, but, if I had been in Lydecker's shoes and felt as strongly against Linda's credentials as she did, I'd want Linda to know it. I'd want her to know why I felt as I did. And, most importantly, since Lydecker had worked with and known her personally and professionally over the period of three quarterly periods, I'd want to leave a trail of corroborative breadcrumbs that, when the time came to write the damned letter, I could retrieve them confidently because I'd shared them with Linda as those crumbs had dropped.

As it was, Professor Lydecker's letter of recommendation came out of the blue like errant Zeros diving into Oahu seventy years after the invasion. Totally unprofessional. I'd blush with shame if it were discovered that I'd written it.

Professor Lydecker is dead now, killed in a two-car accident at a four-way stop in the hinterlands of rural Wisconsin several years ago. I mean no disrespect, nor do I carry anything more away from the "letter" incident than deep professional disappointment. But the trauma to Linda brought on by it lived on. It scarred her growing self-confidence and sense of self. She wouldn't ever forget it, although, unbeknownst to her, it was only the beginning of the crushing professional upheavals she'd experience over the next few years.

No more than two weeks later, a composed Linda received another phone call from a potential employer, this time another Catholic college on the eastern side of the Mississippi in Wisconsin, Viterbo University. Not a very large school, but a pretty little campus located close to the river near downtown La Crosse. They were enthusiastic about interviewing Linda, and Linda arranged to make the five-hour trip from Mankato three days later. I was excited for her, and, because the negative letter had been excised from her dossier and replaced with another, Linda again felt professionally validated. The interview went very well, the faculty and invited students loved her interactive social studies teaching exercise, and, after she'd returned home in mid-evening, she received a call from the department chair congratulating her on being offered the job.

It was July now, leaving little time to waste for us to plan for Linda to live away from home. There was little we could do about that save turning the job down. But they'd captured Linda on the rebound—she felt she had no choice but to take it, she told me, if only to prove wrong the shadow of the elephant in the room that had declared her incompetent.

As for what she'd be leaving behind, there was only Chris.

He was fourteen now, an athletic kid, bright, handsome, a solid young man with an attitude who had entered the most behaviorally risky period of his life. He had lots of friends not necessarily as smart or morally directed as he was, and they were all itching for a little excitement and, perhaps, minor trouble. Linda was worried about leaving him alone with me, and, sad to say, she was right to be so. I wasn't nearly as watchful as I should have been and sometimes found myself out with my own friends drinking more than I should. I promised her that I'd be vigilant, make sure that he was fed, get him to school, pay attention to where he was going, and with whom, and behave myself. Linda ought to have been more worried about me than Chris, but she was guilt-ridden about her choice to live for the year in La Crosse until we'd sorted out the complexity of our living situation.

That, as it turned out, would be the least of her problems.

CHAPTER 5

The Great Two-Headed Disaster

What follows is a most strange story that mirrors Linda's and my agonizing, many years earlier, over whether I should grab the opportunity of a small-paying offer of a full-time faculty position in Indiana or stay home with Linda and Karen and give Linda room for advancing what was on the way to becoming a successful elementary school teaching career. That's where we were again two weeks after the discovery of Lydecker's crushing letter. Linda and I had the same discussion about whether she should take Viterbo's offer and find a place to live close to that campus five hours away from Chris and me or forego her main chance and stay home with us. A tortured one for her.

Now, there are a lot of differences here. Just like me back in 1977, Linda was looking at her first real full-time college-level teaching assignment. But, more than that, she was looking at self-justification, vindication, for what she well might have believed that Lydecker had put her through. Here, without that colossal indictment of her competence in her file, she received the full endorsement of Viterbo's search committee and administration. It was a mutual hug-in. When I drove down to La Crosse with Linda to begin our search for some living space for her, she also had the department chair get the keys to her office, take us with her to look at the rooms she'd be teaching in, and then meet with her department chair to be briefed on her responsibilities.

Chris, whom I'd brought along to make real for him mom's new professional persona and how important it was to her, and I went to the gym to shoot some hoops. Linda gathered us up a couple of hours later to catch some lunch and buy a paper. Though there weren't many rental listings, we found one right away across the river in Le Center, Minnesota, that looked ideal. A friendly older couple met us at the door of a two-story older house with an outside set of stairs leading to the second floor.

That second floor would be all hers--a nice and roomy apartment of four rooms, lots of windows, and, most importantly, providing a view of a quiet tree-lined street in a safe neighborhood. Very reasonably priced, with no lease. We grabbed it then and there.

But our ride back confirmed to us the huge number of miles that would separate us from Linda. Her plan was to drive home every other weekend, while Chris and I would do the same on the other alternate weekends. It all looked great until we began to do it.

The other thing I'd need to do was find Linda a safe, dependable, and comfortable ride. That meant that my rusty collection of ancient cars wouldn't be candidates. A rental was in the offing, and, I reasoned, a big luxury car to wrap around Linda on her long trips. I found just the thing—a '94 Lincoln two-door Mark IV. It had only 20,000 mostly highway rental miles on it, Linda loved it (who wouldn't?), and I signed a two-year lease for what she and I labeled from that moment "the hot rod Lincoln." Lots of money, but she was more than worth the state of mind that big monthly payment would buy us. And it did.

When the gun sounded for the start of fall semester, Linda was all moved in and growing comfortable with her classes. It was amazing seeing the change in her affect once she started teaching at Viterbo. Happy; self-assured; adjusting.

Of course, there were anxieties for her. She had never lived away from me and the kids for longer than a weekend. She was homesick. That didn't take away from the amount of time she was investing in her work; she'd spend more time at school and at home doing her course prep, reading, and paper-grading because we weren't there to distract her. But she missed us, continued to agonize about Chris, how he was doing in school, how football was going, and whether he was staying out of trouble. She did manage to catch one of his games, and she was thrilled when Chris nearly scored a touchdown.

She was also anxious about how Chris was responding to my attempts to play mom and dad for him. Chris didn't accompany me every weekend that I spent visiting Linda—he had lots of invites from his friends for him to sleep over, and, although I wouldn't allow him to stay home all the time (it wouldn't have been right—Chris clearly needed direction, discipline, connection to his mom, and responsibility to a routine), but, when I went down there alone, Linda and I shared the intimacy that she and our relationship needed. Lots of special dinners out. Walks by the river. A renewal of our sexual life.

I and, as far as I could glean from my conversations with Linda, she had no hint of any problems in her job. She enjoyed her courses, she said; she had started a student teacher group that met each week to share their experiences and support each other. She had gotten nothing but support from her department chair, she said, and she exuded confidence.

At Thanksgiving, Karen brought one of her roommates, Riva, home from Bryn Mawr, and Linda decided that she'd drive us in the hot rod Lincoln down the Mississippi past Lake Pepin to the old Anderson Hotel on the river in Wabasha to spend the night, bring in a couple of very cuddly and fat hotel cats to sleep with us, and have a traditional family-style Thanksgiving dinner. Linda was over-the-moon ecstatic. She had her family around her, Riva was a hilarious delight, and we'd all had the best Thanksgiving ever. Linda topped it off on the way home by driving to a viewing spot not far up-river so that we could all look in awe at the huge gathering of eagles at a shoal in the river.

But enter the totally unexpected at the end of the

following week. Before we'd driven Karen and Riva to the airport to finish their semester at Bryn Mawr, Linda had expressed confidence and optimism about her job. Of course, she knew that her appointment had been tenure track, so her job wouldn't be in jeopardy. However, she told me that she understood how she wanted to create a strong record of accomplishment, and she felt that she had done just that so far.

The next weekend she'd be hosting me and Chris. And she had some very bad news. She'd distributed student evaluations the week before Thanksgiving that were collected by a proctor and returned to the department chair. When Linda got a chance to read them, she was shocked. The responses were mixed, with enough bad numbers to skew the results. When we met in her office, she was bereft. This was diametrically opposed to what she had prepared herself to expect. I couldn't believe what she was telling us—I've had bad student evals before, mostly early on in my career. And I understood how every class was different, regardless of how I felt about the subjectivity involved. In my many fixed-term assignments, a bad eval could really put me in a bad place. But Linda's situation was different; she could carefully look at them, learn from them, and apply some changes to the next group of courses she would teach in spring semester.

But that's not the way Linda's situation would work. When, during the final week of fall semester, she met to discuss those evaluations with the department chair, her boss had already made a decision. Linda would not be given a second chance, she was told. Linda was non-plussed. The chair told her that several students had come to her with complaints about Linda's inflexibility in grading. It seems that Linda had insisted from the start, and had included material in all her syllabi to reinforce her insistence, that all the lesson plans, bios, and position papers they'd write for her would need to be carefully edited. She'd also indicated that their work would be graded on the overall quality of their final copies. She was requiring that all her students take full responsibility for what they'd written. Exert editorial control.

For someone like me who'd graded my students' work in the same way, what I saw Linda asking of hers didn't seem unreasonable. But I was in English. From Linda's perspective, students needed to be concerned about their audience—if they didn't become accustomed to applying quality control in their own writing, they'd be setting a bad example for their present and future students. And, if they didn't concern themselves with the structure, grammar, and mechanics of their writing, it's possible that they may not have learned those skills and wouldn't be capable of helping their students master them. And that's what she told the chair.

But, it seems, that wasn't the chair's main concern. Student retention and graduation numbers were. And, in her view, Linda was jeopardizing both. And that's the way the world works at private institutions of higher learning. Without a huge endowment, Viterbo and other Catholic colleges like them are dependent on enrollment, tuition. A precipitous drop in both could jeopardize Viterbo's ability to sustain itself over the long term. With a total of 1600 undergrads, and with a faculty of only four plus a part-timer in the Education Department, it doesn't take a math wizard to see how a downward shift in enrollment in Education courses could impact what the department could offer and whom they could pay to offer them. It makes sense that the department chair was expressing her reliance on student satisfaction with both their teachers and courses as her main determinant on whether Linda, or any other faculty member, should be kept on.

While doing so may, indeed, raise the question of whether prioritizing student satisfaction (i.e., the questionable argument that students were "consumers" and could take their "business" elsewhere if they weren't happy with the "product") could cause teachers to teach down rather than up to their students, Linda was being confronted with an economic reality. Keeping students in their seats rather than providing them reasons to leave or transfer to other colleges was a big deal at a time of higher tuition and a smaller number of applicants for freshman seats.

What was harder to understand was the department's foreclosure of Linda's future at Viterbo so quickly and finally. An unusually (in my experience) quick trigger. Because of one set of bad evaluations, Linda was being handed her walking papers. That kind of quick expression of no confidence has happened where I taught if questions of frequent and unapproved absence, insubordination, moral turpitude, or abuse of students arose and garnered support, but not one set of bad evals. I may have found myself in some jeopardy too if it did. And, of course, there was my first-year dust-up with the dean when, over the phone, I informed her that she should perform an impossible and obscene act upon herself. Three days off, but not for the "go fuck yourself." I worked in a union shop, and, if Linda had, she would have received immediate support and advocacy from union stewards and officers. But she didn't, and they couldn't.

Therefore, Linda was left to twist in the wind. Because she was hired on a tenure track, her department chair couldn't simply end her employment. But she did the next worse thing—a thing that, at the time and even now, I find impossible to understand. Linda, her chair told her, was done. There would be no opportunity for redemption. That is—and Linda pleaded for this opportunity—no improved results of evaluations for her spring courses would save her. Her chair was adamant that, although Linda would be teaching for Viterbo in spring semester—hell, she had already been notified when and what she'd be teaching then, and the schedule of courses and teachers had already been circulated to students in preparation for their registration! — improved evals wouldn't matter, even though she'd be required to administer them.

When Linda pleaded for a chance to study those negative evaluations, discover what students had found deficient in her teaching or student interactions, and then implement changes, the effects of which could be measured in the next set of evals, the chair applauded her but said Linda's situation was irrevocably settled. It was all about the numbers, Linda's were bad, and the die was cast. Yikes! Glad I didn't work there!.

Furthermore (if that weren't enough), Linda would have a decision to make. It is customary, unless the reasons for departure were grave, for anyone working on a tenure-track appointment to be offered a "walk year" if a decision has been made by the administration to cut bait. That is, Linda could accept that additional year of employment to try to do her best work while applying for a new job, if she ever wanted one. That "walk year" would also enable her chair to advertise for a competent person to replace her. But she wouldn't have to.

Imagine what Linda was laboring through here. Try to place yourself in her shoes as she was nearly hyperventilating, trying desperately to absorb what she was being told—that her work in the eyes of her students hadn't been anywhere as good as she had confidently assumed it was. An apparently secure tenure track job going up in smoke. Now you see it; now you don't. Any thoughts of continuing beyond that year into the next had to be colored—or poisoned—by the thought that there'd be students in her future classes who'd dropped the axe on her and colleagues who'd know that she was a dead woman walking.

Well, it was the end of the semester, and she took the time with me and Chris in the security of her home to gather herself emotionally after the shock of rejection and the imputation of not being who she believed she was. We huddled over those bad evals and found that there was one common denominator among them all: her prioritizing of the mechanics of writing and her method of downgrading student work that hadn't nearly been edited. Quality control.

We agreed that Linda had her own audience problem here. Although she'd been accustomed to teaching fifth grade classes of captive students who sat in the same seats throughout each day and hadn't matured to the point of knowing their own minds about what they were being taught and how, Linda's Viterbo students were free agents as well as consumers. They could get up and walk away if they didn't like what their teachers were selling them and could register their complaints accordingly. Linda's students very well could have viewed her attempts to get them to take full responsibility for their own writing—particularly when Linda was penalizing them for their mistakes—as an incursion. Why, they might have thought, she's treating us like fifth graders! Even though Linda hadn't meant to convey that impression, she surely did, which speaks to something very important that I'll get to later.

And, so, Linda needed to commit herself to an approach more in line with her current student audience. It would be ok to tell them that what and how they wrote would always be important and that she'd hold them responsible for it, but she might want to keep hands (and red pen) off their papers except for end comments. Prioritize the content of what they wrote first—after all, if they've got nothing to say in the first place of some import, it makes no sense to evaluate the mechanics of what they did not say.

So, we reached consensus on a couple of things. First, make sure, if possible, to say something positive about what they'd written. Second, make a suggestion or two about how they could improve what they'd written. Third, if there were editorial problems in students' papers, focus on one or two of them but don't overwhelm them with red circles and cross-outs in the body of their papers—that amounts to a kind of violation. And fourth, either give them a grade with the option of re-writing for a better one or don't grade the papers at all—treating them as first drafts that will be graded after being re-submitted. Doing these things might make them feel like fellow professionals receiving advice from a benign editor.

But there was another issue she'd need to address that might make those evaluations seem less like odious instruments of torture and more like learning assessments. The distinction is enormous. There's something final about evaluations: they normally happen once at the tail end of a course, with no opportunity to correct teaching missteps already made. In fact, my sense of teacher evaluations is that they are beauty contests that tend to accent the ugly—the warts and blemishes. An assessment is most frequently a snapshot. It could be administered at any time during a given course—several times, ideally—to measure how things have been going. What's working well? What isn't? What do you think could be done better?

Teacher assessments can provide measurements of anything that occurs in a class—how about that last writing assignment? Did I provide enough clarity and direction in it? Did it seem to connect with the goals of the course? And how about my grading of that assignment? What were the strengths and weaknesses of my comments on it? Did the grade make sense when considering the grading criteria on the syllabus?

We hadn't incorporated the use of learning assessments into Mankato State's Valley Writing Workshop, an across-the-curriculum campus-wide faculty improvement opportunity that several faculty and I conducted every year, when Linda had enrolled in it, but we soon made a very big deal about it. Teacher assessments can be short or frequent, but the key is that they provide a teacher with transparency about what she's doing and how she's doing it with her students while there's still plenty of time to change students' perception of their learning experience.

That's why (1) doing multiple assessments during a course is most beneficial to teachers and students and (2) creating one's own assessment tools and strategies in addition to that formal and computer-driven teacher evaluation at the end of the semester is so much more useful. Doing so makes the evaluation process an organic part of learning in any course and anything but a popularity contest.

Linda could see that, should she have asked students to respond to her method of grading early-on—actually, to anything she'd included in her syllabus! —she'd probably have been able to avert a lot of the negative comments she received. And that's precisely how she approached her classes in the spring: a full and open explanation of her syllabi and the goals she'd articulated in them that she intended to reach by the end of the semester. She changed her approach to grading and implemented assessment tools on three occasions during the course. And the results of her evaluations, although not sterling, were much more positive even though, to Linda's chagrin, they had absolutely no effect on her future at Viterbo. But she'd bounced back attitudinally, felt better about herself, and reached a state of emotional equilibrium.

Of course, a month before her spring courses ended, she'd need to inform her chair about whether she intended to do the "walk year." That meant another trip to the lovely park by the Mississippi to puzzle things out. As we reclined on the grass that warm early April day and ate our lunch, I asked only one question: do you want to do this? Linda was unsure about her answer. She knew that she was a "lame duck," and she felt empty because of that. We talked about what she'd do if she walked away—there was subbing again. There'd always be that. It wasn't too late to apply for other jobs, I told her--after all, she'd landed the Viterbo gig the previous summer after she'd gotten her degree. But she wasn't at all ready for that, she said. In fact, she was unsure whether she wanted to continue to teach at all.

No way for her to go back to elementary school teaching. She'd priced herself out of that possibility with her two advanced degrees. She surely could go home and be queen of the house again; Chris was an incommunicative and surly fifteen now, and, although not a bad kid, hard to manage but still operating on the margins of acceptable social behavior. No problems with the law, but some of his friends continued to be sketchy and he needed watching. I posited that, given the windshield wiper of explosive emotions that Linda had exhibited over the past several months—and understandably so—I could see Linda and Chris at each other's throats at high decibel levels. That had already been the case before Linda left for Viterbo. Teenagers. Alienation. Guaranteed unpleasantness.

At the end of our discussion, Linda decided to do the "walk year." She didn't do so ecstatically. Lots of baggage still to be tripped over. But, true to the person I'd known since she was sixteen, she *couldn't* give up. She couldn't leave Viterbo without showing anyone who cared to look that she was a professional. She still had her apartment in Le Center and a talking cockatiel to keep her company. She found real value in going around La

Crosse and neighboring communities working with cooperating teachers and the student teachers in her charge. She was good at it.

And she had a plan for addressing her classes and students that felt safe and comfortable. She'd continue sponsoring Viterbo's Future Teacher Club and going to regional educational meetings. She said that she wasn't kidding herself, that she still hurt badly from the wounds her meeting and subsequent interactions with her chair had inflicted. And she was realistic about how she may have unintentionally hurt herself with her writing mechanics crusade. Inflexibility. But she still felt, as I did, that Viterbo had pulled the plug on her too soon and, though it might not have mattered to Viterbo, she'd try to vindicate herself and figure out whether she wanted to try again at another university.

Not even with the benefit of hindsight (you'll see what I mean in just a bit), I wished I'd had the guts to talk her out of it. I failed to remind her that, flushed with what she believed was her success in her first couple of months at Viterbo and all the happy exchanges between Linda and the faculty, she had called me at my office with news of an opening in the English Department and how wonderful it would be if we were working together in what neither of us yet recognized as a toxic work environment. It would have been bad news for both of us if I'd been hired to work there at the very moment that Linda was being rejected. Good God!

I couldn't get the Lydecker apocalypse out of my mind or the nagging question of whether Linda was fit for college teaching. And there was more than a little blame on my side for her ending up in the disappointing situation that she was in. "You can do it, Linda! I know what some have told us about how you shouldn't pursue a Ph.D. But this may be your moment! Let's go ahead and prove those folks wrong. Who says you'll never get a university job? I'm behind you all the way." A booster shot that is as true as it was unnecessary, stupid, and selfish.

And look what that had won for her? But, on the cusp of

her taking the "walk year" at Viterbo, some of the most crucial aspects of Linda's psychological reality had not changed. Perhaps some of them had grown worse. Certainly, from the time she was eighteen and determined, as the anonymous narrator in *The Handmaid's Tale* discovered written at the bottom of her closet, not to let the bastards get her down, she was stubborn and pushed back hard when she felt wronged; she got her back up against those that belittled her abilities. She'd show them.

But there was the weight problem. As it had always been, being overweight contributed negatively to Linda's sense of self. She had regained all the weight she'd lost from her fasting diet since her trip to Philadelphia to visit Karen at college. When she took the Viterbo job, she was as heavy as she'd ever been, and she kept that weight on through that first harrowing year in La Crosse. And why wouldn't she? She was living alone, with only intermittent up-close-and-personal support from me when she really needed it. She'd always tended to eat more—I do too! — when lonely or operating under full anxiety, and that was her reality. Disappointment, guilt, and failure were cues to use food as a defense mechanism, I think, a response directly counter to how being extremely heavy made her feel about herself.

It's interesting to speculate on how the intervention of a mental health professional in 1988—particularly a woman whom she felt comfortable confiding in—seems to have led to some of Linda's greatest achievements: losing a huge amount of weight, finishing two advanced degrees, and securing a professional appointment. But, in her semi-isolation, she refused to consider trying to find another psychological sounding board. She needed one desperately. Without it, she'd simply be plowing ahead into her meaningless year at Viterbo without addressing any of the accumulating and highly combustible shocks and traumas that festered inside her. As my wise mom was fond of saying, "the go-ahead boys stuck in the mud." On the surface, she could show the world a sense of calm and control which belied the maelstrom that boiled inside.

She plunged into her final year at Viterbo with her pet

cockatiel—until it found its way out a screen door blown open by the wind—and our bi-weekly visits. And she persevered, poured herself into her teaching, and received good, if not great, evaluation results. To the still open question of whether she would open herself up to failure again and apply for another full-time college teaching position, she paid attention to job notices through the spring and remained noncommittal until a pair of openings at Augsburg College in Minneapolis crossed her desk.

Again, these were jobs that, if her failure at Viterbo hadn't severely bruised her self-confidence, had her name written all over them. A call for a Ph.D. in Curriculum and Instruction with specialties in teaching either science or math or social studies and language arts whose responsibilities would include supervising student teachers in metro schools. Nothing unusual about the ancillary aspects of these jobs—contributing to departmental committees, attending and presenting at conferences, writing articles for publication in regional and national journals. Again, a sectarian institution, one that offered no continuing support for their teachers via a union, but, I reasoned, might be expected to offer such support given the large community of colleges and universities it was situated in and the cosmopolitan atmosphere of the Twin Cities.

If it sounds like I was vaguely rooting for Linda to apply for one of those jobs, you're right. Never mind the maxim that the beatings will continue until morale improves. I wanted Linda to win, whatever I thought winning might look like. And I'm sure that my partiality bled through into her decision-making. But I'd be responsible for what she did no matter how objective I'd pretend to be because I'd put her into this predicament years before by my wrong-headed advocacy. I was that Far Side cartoon pushing the door the wrong way for entrance.

Why couldn't I have left her alone, for Christ's sake, to be her own person? She trusted me, and I betrayed that trust for my own ego repeatedly. I know now—nothing like hindsight—that I should have counselled her (if I counselled her at all)—to walk away from this job opening, and teaching in general, and go ahead and do what she'd always enjoyed most: watching a bad soap opera, making and consigning jewelry, knitting and crocheting and macrame-ing and painting and crewel-ing and photo album-making and being with her kids. Although I don't know for certain, I think Linda applied for that Augsburg job because she thought she'd be letting me down if she didn't. Jesus.

And she got the job. Again, because it was a sectarian private, not for a lot of money. But the place seemed—and this is admittedly biased and judgmental opinion with no real foundation—like a more legitimate institution of higher learning. The student body wasn't appreciably larger than Viterbo's, but they employed more faculty in addressing students' needs. Oh, they were just as paranoid about keeping their consumers happy and retained, as Linda and I would discover in spades when things would horribly blow up there nearly three years down the road. Linda's was a busy little department big enough to hold little get-togethers. There were young as well as mid-career faculty represented in it with a male department chair who legitimately supported his department members and tried to meet their needs.

Linda was happy there from the start in the fall of 1995. She made friends immediately with another young hire and her partner and socialized outside of school while comparing notes as time went by about what the department and college expected from them. Augsburg had—to me—an unusual tenure arrangement that required faculty, three years in, to submit all evidence that supported their appointments being continued for an additional three years up to their tenure year. Actually, without an actual mentoring system in place to ensure that new faculty knew precisely what would be required of them for continuation of their positions, this two-stage approval process left no doubt about what the university wanted to accomplish regularly and how to document it. Good teaching. Attendance at professional meetings. Evidence of some regular professional writing. Evidence of community service.

With purpose, confidence, and a feeling of belonging, Linda set to work. And, over those first three years, she did well.

Her course evaluations were consistently good. She traveled with members of the department to places like Nashville and Dallas to attend conferences. She wrote a short piece, from a personal narrative perspective, on her work as a student teacher supervisor. And she was deeply involved in the work of the department. When Linda and I bought a small cabin on the south side of Lake Superior, we invited a faculty member and her husband to visit us there and had a great time.

There were complications and inconveniences, to be sure. She needed to regularly rent an apartment one or two days each week near Augsburg's campus to make it easier to meet her early morning classes and observe her students teaching in city locations. There was the mind-numbing eighty-mile commute from Mankato and across the cities to get to work. We faced the quandary about needing to move—we nearly bought a new house in Northfield off 35W in late fall of 1997—to get closer to Augsburg while at the same time not disrupting our son Christopher's life as he was about to enter his senior year of high school. But, instead, Linda found her own life radically disrupted a few months later.

Just after Chris' graduation, Linda and I found an inexpensive and workable housing alternative in a Bloomington condo that would gain Linda easier access to Augsburg while opening up car pool options for me several days each week for a straight shot up 169 to Mankato. And then it all fell down.

I'm an ardent believer in chaos theory to account for the way the universe works. Forget about an all-knowing god who knows if you've been bad or good, so be good for goodness' sake. No notion of a universe driven by a sense of moral justice through time. And determinism suggests an order that isn't there. For my money, Lucretius had the answer. Endless atoms ricocheting off one another unpredictably like ping pong balls during the selection of a power ball winner. Chance. Luck. Things just happen without rhyme or reason or pattern. Of course there's free will to choose one's path, but no way to anticipate the crazy events along that path that very well might short-circuit it.

One must humbly be prepared to suffer the slings and arrows of outrageous fortune. Sort of like Sisyphus and his infernal rock. Or, for anyone like me who has used meager skills to build a house single-handed, the frustrating and destructive appearances of "Murphy" to screw up the works.

As near as I can figure it, in the spring of 1998, only a matter of a couple of months before her three-year report was due to be submitted to her department chair, one of those directionless ping pong balls collided with Linda. The event occurred in a mid-weeknight class of one of her curriculum and instruction courses. It doesn't matter which one. The subject is immaterial. Linda had lectured a bit, introduced a problem for her class full of students to solve, and then divided them into small groups to address the problem and devise strategies for dealing with it. Linda had worked with the best practitioners of collaborative learning at the University of Minnesota right down the street from her class. She'd taken the Johnson brothers' theory and practice and built a dissertation around a semester-long research problem for three fifth-grade classes.

As her college student groups worked over twelve to fifteen minutes, Linda walked among them to observe how they were progressing and to answer questions that might clarify their interactions. And, as she was looking closely at the work of one particular group, she'd innocently and inadvertently placed her arm across the shoulders of a female student. I'm sure that she'd done it before in other classes over time, whether it may have involved college-age students or ten-year-olds. But she'd never received the reaction that she did that evening. It was immediately defensive, angry, and loud. In fact, the young woman told Linda, within hearing distance of almost everyone in the class, "Don't touch me!"

Linda immediately apologized to the young woman and told her that she meant nothing by it except as a gesture of support. But the young woman wouldn't accept Linda's apology, continued to take umbrage at what she asserted was an invasion of her personal space, and the upsetting situation continued to unfold.

For her part, Linda acted quickly and professionally. Excusing herself from the class and putting one of her students in momentary charge, she called security, but, when they didn't respond, Linda rushed to the department office looking for someone who could witness and validate what had and would occur. Finding someone not in elementary education but from another area working late, she quickly told the woman what had just happened and asked if she could accompany her to her classroom.

While Linda took scrupulous notes of what each of her students said about the situation and recorded the outlines and key quotes associated with what had happened earlier, particularly from the offended young woman, her witness conducted an interview of those who wished to comment on what had happened, with special emphasis upon the still angry student. After Linda had committed as much information as she could to paper and had the witness sign her notes, there was nothing left to do but to offer her regrets to the class for the classroom disturbance, provide an assignment for the following class, and dismiss them for the evening.

But what had happened that night was just the beginning of what "chance" would wreak on Linda. I'd just arrived home myself after having taught a night class at MSU. As I was preparing a snack and a glass of wine, Linda burst through the door to the garage and up the stairs. She was badly shaken, panicked, and furious at the same time. I listened horrified as she narrated the events of her evening, how she'd tried to protect herself with some anecdotal and evidentiary proof—I applauded her clear and quick thinking. She'd managed to keep it together during the incident, showing only a calm and caring and professional face to her class.

But now she was thoroughly distraught, on the verge of an emotional meltdown. She knew she shouldn't have touched her student—I remember so vividly those classes staged for faculty at MSU several years earlier in which we were educated about the many forms of student harassment that faculty could subject their students to while putting themselves and the university at legal risk. But Linda meant nothing by it; her heart was pure. She was barely conscious of having done it, it being an extension of emotional caring that, she said, had been a part of her interactions among a very large extended Italian family upbringing. It's a shame that Dorothy hadn't shown more of it.

But none of that mattered now as Linda cried bitterly in my arms. She'd need to revisit what she'd just endured all over again the next day in a meeting with her chair. As she'd discover while pouring it all out to him, he was shocked, too. He had received the message from his wife that Linda had tried to reach him the previous evening along with a hurried brief impression of the problem she was grappling with. He listened attentively, extending his support to Linda with the cautionary note that a fuller investigation would need to occur—she had a sense now of the bureaucratic response that would be coming.

I can't imagine the embarrassment and sense of humiliation she must have felt in the following days in sharing with several faculty what had transpired. They were supportive and understanding, but a couple of them warned sympathetically that there would probably be hell to pay. And they were right. The first hell was entering her next night class with the party in question in attendance. And who should be sitting in the back of the room but the angry party's significant other--an angry and self-righteous one, too. In my book, a completely unacceptable situation that I'd had to manage once early in my career. Linda politely asked why he was there, to which he responded, "to protect my girlfriend."

I don't know what I would have done. I know what I wanted to do the next time her class was scheduled to meet when she told me, but my being there would have only been more incendiary and unsupportive, so I desisted. Facing this hostile presence, what could my 5'1" little spouse have been thinking and feeling during that interaction? Inchoate terror, perhaps. But, always the pro, she offered the man an opportunity to stay as long as he did not disturb or disrupt the class; but, if he did, she'd call security. And he behaved, while glowering at her the whole time.

In the following days and weeks, Linda's dignity and self-control would need to survive two meetings. The first would be an explanatory departmental meeting concerning the upheaval that had occurred in her class and how she had handled it. During that meeting she received support from her chair and the faculty person who Linda asked to intervene for her; but a departmental decision on the situation would have to wait until Linda had her second meeting that would focus on her renewal with the college dean and the renewal committee.

The department chair would be included in the meeting, but, while he commiserated with the vulnerability of her situation and indicated that he'd advocate for her, because he hadn't been present on the scene, the dean said, his word wouldn't avail much. The girl in question attended the meeting as well, and her story and accusatory tone hadn't changed. After the girl was ushered out of the meeting, another faculty and the dean questioned why she had "put her hands" on the woman, and how she didn't seem to understand that she ought to have known better than to do so. Of course, the dean said, they'd have to accept the word of the student, whether she had misread Linda's intention or not. There were potential liability issues for the university, he said.

Linda, up to that point, had managed her emotions admirably. But, after that, with no one in her corner actively advocating for her, she broke down and cried. Later on after she'd returned home and recalled this emotional climax of the meeting, she said that she felt doubly violated. Not only did the committee take the word of a student over hers, but she felt the shame of her professional demeanor shattering by crying in front of them.

There will likely be a special place in my beloved Dante's hell for me—perhaps the circle of the false counsellors. No question.

CHAPTER 6

It's [Nearly] All Over Now, Baby Blue
--Bob Dylan

And this was finally where all these traumas had been heading: whereas I, some thirty-five years earlier had suffered, among other things, a severe concussion from being in a car that collided head-on with a tree at 90, Linda's concussive collision at Augsburg would inflict greater, longer-lasting injury.

After another devastating, humiliating "walk" year that she was encouraged to take by her department chair, on her part because, within the mental confusion that the incident at Augsburg had wrought, she still held on to the remote possibility that her teaching career wasn't done. In fact, she was invited to interview at St. Kate's in St. Paul, with (as she reported to me with some enthusiasm) success from her public presentation of a science lesson for kids—again, she came in second in that search.

But she was, in fact, done. All the positivity that she had brought to her classroom teaching since 1967 had evaporated. I'm sure that Linda held on for that curtain call at Augsburg as an expression of her dignity. Karen would be getting married in July of 1999. Although she knew that she would have lost nothing in her daughter's eyes—there was no one more supportive of

Linda nor understanding, both during her continuing struggles to establish herself in a college teaching career as well as during the next twenty-three years where we both agonized and compassionated over the steady erosion of Linda's mental and physical condition—Linda wanted to play a large part in Karen's marital preparations.

And she was involved in every part of it, including visiting all the potential venues for the outdoor ceremony and providing advice; evaluating the several sites for the reception, including actually eating the food that these places would offer; and accompanying Karen to bridal stores to help her decide on her dress (in the end, Linda would take charge of actually making important changes to the dress that Karen chose with magnificent effect).

But, as locked at the hip with Karen as she was in the wedding prep, one must understand that I'd run away with Linda to a justice of the peace, furtively married her, denied her what I think she'd always hoped for, a public church wedding and reception gala. Even though I had acceded in 1990 on our twenty-fifth wedding anniversary to do a full-dress renewal of our vows before a priest and friend—the very priest whom Linda had tracked down to preside over Karen and Hunter's wedding—I don't believe Linda had confided to Karen in a full and open way what had happened to her at Augsburg and what she was still living through. She desperately wanted her daughter to be proud of her. So, she put on an enthusiastic, joyful face through that entire year, living, essentially, a double life. And, when the wedding was over and the bridal couple had escaped to their idyllic honeymoon in Bali, the residual effects of the impact of the collision at Augsburg had just begun.

Even though neither Linda nor I knew it, that crash was a cumulative one, inflated beyond its singular effects to include all of the many mental shocks that had occurred throughout her life, each one of which had been allowed to go untreated, unaddressed, before the next shock, and the next, and the next, came along to compound the effects of the previous one. I remember encountering for the first time Dylan Thomas' wonderful little memoir "Memories of Christmas" in the early '80s and teaching it to my students. At one point, Thomas compares his recollective process to compacting a snowball at the top of a hill and then letting it roll down, watching it accrete as it gains speed until it becomes a gigantic tumbling mass, each inchoate snowflake comprising it representing a single memory.

The metaphor seems to fit Linda here. No sustained thought had been given, by her or me, to addressing each one of those mental snowflakes as they occurred. There were no time delays between each of the traumatic events in her life, no pause to slow the speed by which the cumulating snowball of traumas had accreted into an avalanche. And, once again, at the end of the summer of 1999, she had elected fiercely to keep the last one of the many to herself, to suppress, to repress, while letting those earlier traumatic events fade into a blur. A bit later in this narrative, I'll need an assist from Bessel van der Kolk's book about the indelible record of shocks and traumas that, over time, Linda's body kept.

By then, Linda had already begun to show cerebral cracks that suggested an inevitable weakening in her defenses. And, in fact, when dementia starts, defenses melt away. I've already indicated two important things about Linda's emotional make-up that could have made her more vulnerable to that weakening. One of them, outward displays of warmth, caring, and affection, had initially drawn me to her but also had brought about her painful dismissal from Augsburg. She couldn't help expressing them; they were as natural to her as smiling or scratching an itch. This wasn't the former governor of New York, Cuomo, for Christ's sake, self-justifying not being able to keep his hands off nearly all young attractive women within his immediate sphere of influence. And it wasn't any male predator operating opportunistically before or amid the "me-too" movement. It was a woman who used her hands and entire body to communicate her care and protection of those in her charge. I'd seen it repeatedly in my own life, and inside the classes of children that she had taught.

But the second was rage. Linda had always, as I've described from her childhood years, been capable of expressions of extreme anger. A formidable, explosive temper. Linda had always been a person who wore her emotions on her sleeve. One could always tell just by looking at her face or reading her body language—except for those times when she was fully immersed in her role as teaching professional—how she felt, what she was feeling, whether she was running hot or cold. There was really no "off" button on her emotions. She wore them like a billboard. I've always loved that about her. No hiding. No pretenses. Just Linda, out-front and transparent. Chalk that up to her Italian heritage, she used to tell me, although doing so would inevitably lead one into the old stereotypical trap.

Luckily, for the greatest proportion of our relationship, we fought hard but fairly, rarely getting angry at each other at the same time. And that was a good thing because, when Linda was angry, she was furious. Never an in-between. Full-on. And, just as quickly, the dark clouds would pass. A roller coaster of emotions.

By comparison, it had always seemed strange to me that Linda's mother presented an extremely passive affect, although Linda would correct my misapprehension. "She's putting on an act," she said. "She wants everyone to think that she is cultured and educated and, most certainly, she's playing for their attention." But, when there were no outsiders to impress, Dorothy could be mean, spiteful, and, when Linda was young, the wielder of instruments of pain to inflict corporal punishment on her. Lots of frustration and disappointment felt by the widow on the corner with two kids who wanted so much more than she had and struck out at Linda to release it.

I had started to see more of that fury—rage--in Linda's behavior during the '90s. Some of that rage burned as an expression of paranoia. A new faculty member and his wife, having just bought a house in the neighborhood, had brought their son along to interact with Chris while the four of us chatted in the living room upstairs. At the end of the evening after they'd left for home, Linda had wandered into Chris' downstairs bedroom and noticed that a personal article of his was apparently missing. She was sure of it—but she was even more sure that the young man who had accompanied his parents had walked off with it. I believe it was a watch of very little value, but the object's identity doesn't matter. So certain was she of the young man's guilt that she was on the phone to the parents immediately, hardly leaving enough time for them to walk the two streets to their house. Linda's tone was sharp and accusatory; the confused mom on the other end of the line, having queried her son, was just as certain that he hadn't done anything wrong.

Linda hung up angrily, laying waste to the relaxed and friendly evening we'd spent with them, and marched down to Chris' room to search frenetically again. And, after a while, we found it lying under some soiled clothing behind Chris' chest of drawers. Ouch. Linda called the mom back the next day to apologize, but Linda's voice was strained and unconvincing. The friendship was over before it had barely begun. And I remember feeling as if I was teetering on a knife's edge in talking to her about it.

That scene repeated itself, certainly in her souring relationship with my son, but also with one of her best friends—I'll call her Franny. Almost from the first day of my employment at MSU, Linda and I had been fast and steady friends with Franny, her husband and my colleague, and their three lovely and admirable children. We shared years of Thanksgiving and Easter dinners; we spent quality time at their cabin with their extended family in northern Wisconsin. Her husband was a brilliant teacher and leader, and, even though he could be perceived as distant and guarded, he became warmer and more supportive the longer one knew him. Same with their kids—wonderful human beings whom I loved like my own. Linda made it standard practice to have lunch with Franny once or twice each week while she was employed at the university as a student teacher supervisor, and it had gone well for a while.

But soon, as proud parents are wont to do, Franny exuded over the successes and accomplishments of her kids—their prowess in sports, their academic achievements, their ability to gain acceptance to the private colleges and universities of their choice. Before long, the exuding ignited a low-grade competition, and, when I got home from work, I received an increasingly loud and angry play-by-play of who won lunch that day. Now, there's a certain amount of tone-deafness at play when a couple of proud mothers, but good friends just the same, effusively celebrate their kids to each other. And the competition escalated.

Linda, to some extent, felt disadvantaged—poor Chris' uneven performance in high school, including getting kicked off the golf team for being caught smoking and a generally challenging attitude, even while Karen was holding her own in her first year at Bryn Mawr. But the more the uneven competition continued, the angrier and more frustrated Linda became, not a gleaming recipe for a healthy friendship. She should have let it all wash over her, but that's easy for me to say. For her part, Franny should have taken a time-out to listen to herself.

Meanwhile, I became the dumping ground of the deafening angry recitations of what happened that day at lunch. Until they stopped, as did the lunches. We didn't have Easter dinner at Franny's house that year, and forever more. I remember Linda making a call to Franny at the very last minute to pull the plug on our attendance along with the food that we'd agreed to bring and share. Awkward.

Linda simmered over the endgame of her relationship with Franny and her family. Decades later near the end of my time at MSU, I walked down the hall in mid-evening and passed the open-doored office that Franny had been using while teaching an adjunct course. And there she was. I said hello; she lied politely about how good I looked, and then asked me "what happened, Bill, to us, our friendship, and our family interactions? What went wrong?" I told her that I didn't know. But, of course, I did.

And that was the last word I spoke to her or her family

until a few days after Linda died on March 20, 2022, to respectfully inform them of her passing, given how many good miles we'd put on our friendship so many years ago. And once more, she asked me, "What went wrong with us?" This time, I told her that I knew, and, when she pushed me to expand, I demurred, saying that sometime in the future, over coffee, I'd save that explanation for then. Not a chance in this world or the next.

That temper expressed itself increasingly after Augsburg. Lots of reasons for it, I'm certain, but it had always been there. From the first time I'd felt the brunt of it early in our relationship, I'd known better than to interrupt or reason her through it. Whether it was accompanied by flying objects, door-slammings, and martial stompings as the decibel level of her profane shouts rose, I knew enough to let it pass like a violent thunderstorm. And it always had. A generally short shelf-life, after which tears flowed and mutual apologies followed.

There was that time in my university office some fifteen years after I'd quit smoking, but only officially since I'd been regularly "borrowing" cigarettes from my students and furtively secreting a pack in one of my desk drawers along with a lighter and a handy ashtray. Linda was working for the university at that time and happened to come down from the floor above to invite me to lunch. I had left my office door open as I always had, providing Linda carte blanche to discover where the noxious smell of smoke emanated from. When I returned, I could tell that she'd been there by the trail of wreckage she'd left behind. After she'd found the cigarettes, she'd literally shredded them all over my desk and office floor and done the same with the half-full ashtray. And, from the noise and singularly angry voice my adjoining office occupants had reported to me, she had made her rageful presence known.

There had been many of these in our relationship, most not nearly as public or violent as this one. But, after Augsburg, they could occur at any time, and not always directed at me. Perhaps the most disturbing of them occurred around 2001. This time, though, the object of Linda's rage was another of her best friends. Every day, for years, Melissa (not her real name) and Linda would walk together for an hour in and around the neighborhood. Melissa was a tenured professor at MSU; she and her husband lived only a couple of blocks away. I wasn't a big fan of Melissa, and Linda knew that. Melissa was a needy woman, overly self-concerned, very much dependent on a husband, also employed at the university, who seemed less than regardful of the love that Melissa had for him. She mostly chatted aimlessly about others and about what she perceived as her physical imperfections and how she might correct them.

For Linda's part, she just enjoyed the company of another, getting some exercise, and having the opportunity to talk about something other than kids because, well into her middle years, Melissa had none. She and her husband had welcomed us and our kids to their cabin in the Arrowhead on the Big Lake, and we reciprocated a couple of years later by hosting her visit to our cabin for several days. Over the years they became good friends, so good, in fact, that Karen, understanding their closeness and at Linda's behest, extended her an invitation to her wedding in 1999. Both Linda and Karen were less than impressed by Melissa's wedding gift of a small stuffed animal; it might have been better if she'd brought no gift at all, but Linda thought little of it, chalking off that inappropriate gift as typical of Melissa's unintended but real thoughtlessness.

A couple of years after the Augsburg fiasco, Melissa called to tell Linda that she'd be driving down to the Cities to do some shopping and asked her if they could arrange to have lunch. By that time, Linda had found a job creating websites for a new company called Techies.com that specialized in advertising job openings digitally to tech professionals. Her place of employment was located a mere three-quarters of a mile from our condo; although Linda had only a half hour for lunch, she said that they could have lunch at our place if Melissa could arrive a bit early so that they could maximize their time together. Agreeing on the time and date, they rung off.

But Linda hadn't figured on Melissa's frequent negligence about details and her penchant for tardiness. That was true even regarding her lateness to Karen's outdoor wedding ceremony. When the date for their luncheon arrived, Linda raced home, made soup and sandwiches, and waited for Melissa to arrive. And waited. And waited.

Just before 12:30, as Linda was getting ready to return to work, Melissa ascended our back porch stairs. Linda was livid. "Where have you been? I told you that my lunch break is short," she simmered. In typically negligent fashion, Melissa tried to calm her by saying, "Oh, don't worry about it, Linda, I'm sure they'll cut you some slack. Sorry I'm late. A couple of students pushed my office hours longer than I expected." But Linda was on fire by now: "Why couldn't you have called me or sent an e-mail that you'd be late? We could have done it another time. But, as it is, you've left me flat with a bunch of uneaten food." And then a completely tone-deaf Melissa applied the coup de grace: "I don't understand what you're so mad about."

And that did it. Linda erupted all over her like Vesuvius. The loudness of the explosion would have been audible from our back porch to any neighbor near an open or closed window. Linda verbally hit her squarely in the face with her insensitivity and lack of consideration, but it was worse than that. It was a bridge-burning. Linda told me later, still white hot from the encounter, that she screamed "from this point forward, we are no longer friends. I have no respect for anyone who can show none to me. Get out and let me get back to my job. I don't want to see you again."

Pretty violent and painful, to be sure. But, to provide a more vivid sense of how impactful, how traumatic this public rejection was to Melissa, I need to flash forward seven years to 2008. As I was walking quickly and with head down from the building I worked in through an archway into the next on my way to grab lunch and bring it back to my office, I nearly ran headlong into Melissa. The incident between Linda and Melissa hardly registered in my mind when I offered a friendly greeting and asked how she'd been—what a semi-conscious jerk I was!

The halls were crowded with students and faculty, but from that moment until the end of our interaction I became unaware of anyone except Melissa. She reacted to my greeting as if I'd wounded her with a knife. She wrapped her arms around her body as if defending herself from still another blow I might deliver. When I asked her what was wrong, she began to cry quietly.

As we walked clumsily down the hall, Melissa mumbling incoherently all the way, I became aware that we'd begun to attract considerable attention from passers-by, two who were faculty whom I didn't know but who I discovered later worked with her. As Melissa continued to cry, one of the faculty members attempted to intercede on her behalf, not directing his words to me but to Melissa with the strong hint that I'd done or said something just now to hurt or abuse her.

As we neared the cafeteria, I made a critical and stupid miscalculation. Finally gleaning (what a mental giant am I!) that Melissa's near collapse had to do with the violent end to her friendship with Linda, I tried to comfort her with the following words: "I'm sure that Linda didn't mean what she said. She was just under a lot of work pressure. You two were such good friends—I'll bet she'd love to hear from you. Why don't you give her a call?"

I discovered just how mindless and inept my attempt to console Melissa was when she broke into full-blown blubbering. As her faculty friend tried to comfort her, she blurted out to me loudly, "There's something terribly wrong with Linda. I feel so sorry for you to have to continue living with someone as mentally ill as she is! I can't imagine what she's done to you!" To which I paid my respects and beat a hasty retreat. Pure public humiliation.

Later when I got home, I gently confronted Linda with the details of the scene I'd played a part in. But I was nonplussed by Linda's response: "She had it coming." Linda was still simmering. No hint of remorse. Still burning hot. Maybe just a hint of satisfaction. She hadn't forgotten any of it, hadn't let it go.

And I felt bad for her because of that.

After her all but literal firing and embarrassing exit from Augsburg, the effects of her experience weren't all bad. On the good side, she was out of there, distanced from the field of her humiliation. She was home with a now-married daughter that we could visit in her new home in Michigan. Her son was safely ensconced in the Law Enforcement program at MSU after an almost lost and unfortunate year at Rensselaer Poly in upstate New York, barely escaping with his health after a bad pledging experience, and he was finally doing what he wanted. Linda was seeing her kids fairly settled, happy, and directed.

That left Linda and I with the chance to do some serious and loving bonding, part of which had translated two years later into a family trip to Italy. A wonderful time, right in Linda's ethnic wheelhouse. As was the second trip to Italy, a few years later, when we landed in Rome, slept on rock-hard cots at a little monastery and walked everywhere in the ancient city from the Palatine ruins to the Colosseum to the Jewish quarter, the Trevi Fountain, the Spanish steps, and everything in between. Afterwards, we rented a car, hit all of the Tuscan mountain towns on the way to Cortona, including my getting thrown in jail for ten minutes in Montepulciano for parking in a forbidden zone and disputing the extortionate ticket. Wonderful stuff, including doing what Linda loved most—eating wonderful Italian food everywhere we went. I hadn't seen Linda this happy and engaged in what we were doing since before she took the Viterbo job.

But then it was back to reality. Linda had felt strongly about doing something instead of just sitting around. That meant finding another job outside of teaching. There was an opening for a program writer for an educational software concern just down the street. When she interviewed but didn't get it, she found an online ad for a job with a new little company named Techies that created websites for companies seeking to hire tech professionals. Right up Linda's alley—finally, an opportunity to use her M.S.-Tech degree. And she got it. She may have been the company's oldest employee amid a flock of newly minted young grads who were filled with energy, played basketball and other games during their breaks in what I viewed as a permissive work environment, and bonded with Linda. She enjoyed the job; she was challenged by the work in a good way, made to feel welcome, and it wasn't teaching. But, after about six months there, storm clouds were gathering. This was a time when many aggressive new start-ups attempted to go public, and, unfortunately, Techies' attempt failed, costing Linda her job.

After a short time, she landed a job with Mesaba Airlines, a small regional carrier now defunct, writing up rules, regulations, and job procedures, along with doing some scheduling. Before the company folded, Linda took advantage of one of its few perks to fly us to Detroit to see Karen, Hunter, and newly born Talia for $25 each. Soon, she again found work just a few miles away at a division of BI-Worldwide that assembled rewards packages and excursions for companies who wished to incentivize their employees. Not much stimulation for Linda here, and soon, when cut backs came, Linda, being the last in, was first to go.

And, finally, for two short, grueling weeks, Linda endured working in a cubicle in a large windowless room filled with people doing what she was doing—word processing and editing copywrite materials for insurance companies with a half-hour lunch and two strictly metered fifteen-minute breaks per day. The company that paid her might just as well have had their workers do their work on individual treadmills. Mindless, depressing work, particularly for a person mired in an endless depression. And that concluded the work-related part of Linda's program.

It had become evident that Linda was steadily going downhill now. Physically and mentally. Slowing down. Getting quiet. This once effervescent and voluble woman filled with creative energy increasingly kept her own counsel. Harder and harder to engage her in meaningful conversation, particularly when it had to do with how she was feeling, what she was thinking, and what we could do to make her happy. She was still actively using her hands and mind to create things—I'd set her up with an art table on the second floor of the new carriage house

I'd built at the cabin, where she'd pull herself up the steep outside stairs to make earrings and necklaces out of her endless supply of colorful beads and stones to sell on consignment at a little shop a few miles away.

But she was becoming a strange mix of Dickens' Dr. Manette working silently at his last in the Bastille and a high school kid responding with "fine" when asked by a parent how school had gone. Depression. She was deeply inside, and, if pressed to come out, she'd become angry. Her decision-making facility, once so much a part of who she was in taking charge of family business and entertainment choices, had disappeared. "Whatever you want to do" was her stock unanimated response to questions about where we might go to dinner, what movie to see, or where we might travel.

In just a few more years, what was becoming a kind of emotional blankness would devolve into total disengagement, a silence that became difficult to pierce, an apathetic detachment that would make me feel like I was living with a stranger. I vividly remember the visits we made to Karen and Hunter's newly built home on a lovely sylvan setting overlooking a sheltered lake after they'd moved back to Minnesota. The house was literally a work of art in its number and size of windows and spaciousness, and Linda spoke of it with warmth. But so often Linda would sit silently in a big butterfly chair with hassock while the rest of the family was engaged with other things and stare into space. Linda had been an inveterate reader, ploughing through volumes of challenging pieces of fiction and non-fiction. But she'd be quitting her book club soon when she confided to me that she was finding it increasingly difficult to retain what she had been reading,

Her downhill trajectory was hastened by a chance misstep while preparing to do some food shopping at Cub one January day. Temperatures had been frigid, and, though there was no snow on the ground where Linda parked her car, there was black ice. As Linda swung the heavy door of her old Buick open and put her left foot on pavement to begin to pull herself out of the car, her foot slipped on a patch of black ice and something popped. Pain.

Later, she'd tell me that the pain in her left knee was unbearable. It was on the right side of the knee, and, after a trip to the knee doctor, it was determined that she'd need a replacement. Before she left the office, a cortisone shot was administered by a nurse. A long needle was sent directly into her knee, and Linda screamed with pain. There's nothing wrong with anyone who has a low threshold for pain (each person has her own), and that was Linda. She could barely endure the inflating arm wrap of a blood pressure test, and so this injection was awful for her.

And that's the way things continued to go after her knee replacement in the late summer of 2010. To make matters worse, the pain didn't relent for her after surgery. At least, that was her perception, and, frankly, if that's what she felt, it was real to her. It was soon determined that she'd need to replace the other knee, and the pain-driven hits just kept coming. She wasn't good with her rehab. Her heart wasn't it. Her weight interfered with her ability to make the most of her rehab appointments, to do the bike, to do the things necessary to increase flexion, improve her mobility, and gain back minimal strength. By the point of her second knee op in spring of 2013, she'd become physically inactive and unmotivated to be more so. Because she couldn't push through the discomfort to do the necessary hard work for a full recovery, she'd soon be stuck with two bad new knees that caused her nearly constant pain.

One thing that had always rung Linda's bell had been travel. She had loved the five-week trip we'd taken as a young family to the British Isles in 1988 after the last of several procedures to reconstruct my right leg. Chris could have done without the cathedrals we visited along our 3200-mile driving journey, but he and we loved everything else—occasionally being horrified by my finding myself driving on the wrong side of the road; floating on the Thames up to Hampton Court and down to the Cuttysark and Greenwich; walking all over Hampstead and

Hyde Park; the prospect of the Atlantic from our accommodation at the old Lloyds of London signal house used by Marconi to test his wireless theories; Glastonbury and the Tor, with the roar of low-flying Tornado fighters over our heads; Tintern Abbey on the Wye and the cloud-enveloped Mt. Snowden; the treks among the gorgeous villages of the Lake District; and the lochs and mountains of the Highlands.

Linda and I would return a year and a half later to London and York for our twenty-fifth wedding anniversary trip, during which, at the height of a dangerous flu outbreak, I passed out ill on a jammed tube train at the height of rush hour (I could barely reach the floor because the passengers were pressed so tightly against one another). Linda and I experienced English Christmas magic when the train was held for a full ten minutes with the door open and without one dissenting sound from the passengers until, outside the train and seated with Linda next to me, the conductors had made the determination that I was, in fact, well enough to make my way with Linda's help to the surface. More magic from the front row of a theatre just above Trafalgar Square as we were close enough to catch the flying sweat and spit of Richard Harris playing Pirandello's Henry IV the day after Linda had to actively canvas theatre entrants in order to sell tickets that we couldn't use because I was recovering from my sudden illness—now that was the real, bold, take-charge Linda I had always known and loved!

There were the many family road trips we'd enthusiastically taken with our tag-along camper across the states and through the length and breadth of Canada that provided so many unforgettable stories lovingly retold (did you really get struck with lightning, Bill?; remember when you ran the car out of water, causing you to beg a garage owner to let you use his valve compressor to rebuild a head and replace a blown head gasket while we were enjoying the company of strangers at that camper park a few miles away?).

With all those happy miles and memorable experiences logged over so many years, perhaps I could be forgiven for thinking that it was a depressive funk (it wasn't) that Linda was mired in and that the surest way out of it was to plan more excursions (or forced marches) for her to enjoy with me. "Forgiven?"—we'll soon see.

My first sally into testing my notion that more travel to sunny climes would lift Linda out of her deepening depression occurred as a direct consequence of my third and last sabbatical in the winter of 2010. My plan for my semester leave was (1) to enroll in a rudimentary Italian language course to prepare me (2) to take up residence in the beautiful little hilltop town of Cortona for the purpose of expanding my language-learning in the classroom for direct application to practical interactions in the community in order to prepare me (3) to visit and study and create a visual record of ancient Greek and Roman ruins from Cortona and Rome south to Paestum, Siracusa, Agrigento, and Palermo that I could fold into my Humanities courses. This third objective would force me to use my newly acquired language skills to arrange train travel, accommodations, and restaurant visits (Sicily truly requires the use of Italian; that's true the farther one travels south of Sorrento), seek directions, read essential material germane to the sites I'd be visiting, and conduct regular social interactions.

I'd also need to be ready for strenuous walks over substantial distances and varying terrain. In neither Tuscany nor in points south was there any regard for accessibility. I'd be made to remember that with every step Linda would take and every train she would need to board quickly. But I wasn't thinking of that when I was planning the trip. That says everything one needs to know about me and what I've come to recognize as my special brand of narcissism.

Questions about whether I should have bought her a plane ticket at all faded as I considered how little I could bear to be without her for five weeks from the end of March to the first week of May. And I thought even less about what this trip might cost her physically—she wouldn't have her first knee done until the beginning of August—as soon as she, in the company of

Karen, enrolled at a private language institute in Minneapolis that winter to study Italian with me. What a rollicking, belly-laughing time we had! Karen had always been the linguist among us, but we all struggled mightily to get a footing in the basics. It was just the three of us in that little classroom, led by a friendly young man who bore up under our gaffs, Italian malapropisms, and foolishness.

Linda had a grand time, regardless of our struggles with the language and with the slush and snow we needed to endure to get there. Although Karen had paid more attention than I had to Linda's steadily eroding mental and, particularly, physical difficulties enough to warn me that I should seriously reconsider bringing her along, I paid insufficient heed. There'd also be luggage to carry, stairs to climb, treacherously uneven surfaces, and it might be cold.

It was bad news from the start. The plane ride to from Minneapolis to Rome is a long one, especially if one isn't traveling first class. And the time change is murder. Lots of struggles making myself clear about the train tickets we needed to get to Cortona, and lots of walking to get to the platform from which our train would leave. Boarding that first train was when I began to fully understand what Linda would be up against. Very high and steep steps requiring balance and strength to pull oneself up. Physical difficulties getting to our seats. And, when we gingerly deboarded at the little Cortona station, we found it cold and lonely—no cabs waiting, wind blowing as we looked across the street at the steep and circuitous road that led to the top of the little mountain on which Cortona sat.

Finally, a cab arrived and took us to the city wall gates. After some bad attempts to communicate our need for directions to the tobacco shop, we found it, were given the keys to our pensione, were told that it was only "one street up," and Linda, with only a cane, and I, with our luggage, struggled to the point at which the street we were looking for could be accessed. And, through a narrow alley way, looking decidedly "up," we saw what we had won: a set of wide concrete steps, nearly one hundred of them, leading upwards and opening on the little road by which we could walk another fifty yards to the entrance to our accommodation.

But we weren't done yet. There were still thirty steps to climb to our second-floor pensione. I was blown from our vertical journey, but nothing compared to Linda who was forced to stop many times before she reached the top of that first set of steep stairs. And did I mention that it was cold?

This was never going to do. We'd be residing in this little pensione (and it was, in fact, lovely and well-equipped) for a full three weeks. For her part, Linda's legs held up enough to make that climb several more times, walk with me over every inch of the little city, its cathedral, and museums, dine at every restaurant in the city (the fabulous food kept Linda going), attend an olive oil tasting, and join with me and our classmates in a tagliatelle cooking lesson and wonderful meal with the family who'd taught us. But, except for each step of that long staircase, there wasn't a single flat spot in the entire city that she could find some comfort in.

Almost at the end of those first two weeks, I emailed Karen that, from what I gleaned as a growing sense of disorientation and silence from Linda and the pain that she was obviously feeling, I was strongly considering sending her home on the next plane. And Karen agreed, offering to take Linda in for the balance of the time I'd be absent. But I permitted her to overrule me.

The most life I'd seen from her since we'd arrived in Cortona exploded on me when I stated my intention. "I'm not going anywhere," she shouted. "I can do it. All you need to do is give me some extra time, some rest stops." To my concerns about her safety and health, she stuck her chin out and averred, "I know what I can and can't do (she didn't, of course). I'll let you know when I can't. I'm staying." No way I should have let her get away with it; hell, I was assertive enough to include her in the trip when I shouldn't have and to have reserved a spot for her on the plane, but I was too weak and indecisive to pull the plug on her.

And, so, off we went south on the journey to hell. I should be shot for what I did to her when we prepared to make a train change at the dizzyingly sprawling station complex in Rome. I bought our tickets, but, when Linda decided to make her own way to the platform (our connection would be leaving in a scant thirty minutes, and, since Mussolini, the trains are nearly always on time) without telling me, I panicked. I discovered just how bad my grasp of Italian was when, after feverishly looking everywhere for the platform that matched my ticket, I finally wandered into the station's policia office, where, in describing Linda's physical characteristics, I threw the two cops into total confusion.

After a fashion, they agreed to send a couple of agents out to look for a bad approximation of the person I'd described; eventually, when they returned with no success, I told them about her physical infirmity, her cane, and her instability and convinced them to message her on the station's loudspeaker. Much to my embarrassment, one of the cops and I finally found her, just where she said she'd be, much farther down the very long platform that I'd failed to walk to the end of, totally miffed that I'd taken so long to arrive that we'd missed our train. Total malpractice in the care-taking job I'd assumed with Linda.

Shortly, we boarded another train toward Naples and Sorrento, where Linda put more miles on her aching legs through Herculaneum, but her exertion there was nothing compared to what I'd let her in for as we continued south. Paestum was a huge, marvelous site of an ancient Greek city replete with temples and a community of ruined homes. To get to it after leaving the train, we had to walk a mile and a half up a dirt road before we were picked up by a smiling old man in a little truck who carried us the rest of the way. There was no quit in Linda then or the next day, no matter how tired or lame she was. We made the full circuit of the beautiful site with a few rest breaks, bought a gelato, and Linda was truly thrilled by all of it.

And then it was back on the train to cross the strait at Messina on our journey to an even more impressive city of Greek ruins, the Valley of the Temples, at Agrigento south of Sicily by the sea. Again, the walking over hilly stone and sand-covered paths couldn't have been more difficult for her, unless it was the walk to the head of a steep hill above the ruins to our bed and breakfast accommodation.

In another two days we'd move on southeastward to Siracusa, another serious walking challenge to a nearly worn-out Linda. Lots of acreage to walk over in the huge Archeological Park containing an enormous ancient Greek theatre in the process of readying a production of Oedipus as we struggled over and up its steep and rough rock-hewn stairways to view a stage rehearsal. But there was so much more walking beyond the theatre and into a vast ancient quarry, the primary feature of which was the "ear of Dionysius," an ear-shaped holding cell for prisoners carved deep into the rock. The next day, Linda was nearly done in by the walk to the train station, where, with the aid of two attentive young Tunisian immigrants, Linda was able to board the train for Palermo.

But there was more strenuous walking ahead. After we walked from the stazione centrale about three-quarters of a mile and three flights up steel stairways because the elevator was out of service, we discovered that our reserved accommodation had, in fact, been given away. Back again on the street after a bone-aching stair descent, I sat Linda in an outdoor café while I proceeded up the street in search of an affordable hotel. After another half-mile and a couple of failed attempts, I found, about a block from the main thoroughfare, a full-service hotel whose reservationist happily engaged my bad Italian and, after I retrieved Linda and returned ever so slowly, was able to offer us an excellent, spacious room.

Two days later, there was still the mile and a quarter walk to the station which I did at double-time after placing Linda and our luggage in a cab. And all that was left for us to do was to endure our long train passage back to Rome and the long walk through the station to our final overnight hotel stay before boarding our plane home. Three long, sometimes harrowing, but always painfully exhausting weeks of train travel and walking on uneven surfaces for Linda. I'm ashamed that I put her through it, but, although my daughter will never forgive me for submitting her mother to that ordeal, Linda, after some time to recoup, was thrilled by what she'd experienced. That's no excuse.

But I hadn't learned my lesson. Linda, thanks to me, had eight more years of travel to a variety of venues. There'd be the annual week-long fall pilgrimages to Ogunquit to the most beautiful beach in the world, where we'd meet my sister Penny and her husband Jim, walk the town's roads and beach and area environmental paths, consume as many lobsters and clams as we could (that was Linda's favorite part), and even play some hideous golf with Linda driving one of the golf carts.

I was pushing Linda in a wheelchair by then, and, of course, as I always would, I'd jeopardize Linda's safety by pushing that wheelchair up and down steep paths bordering a fenceless drop to the ocean below. Crazy. My persistent brand of narcissism. Beyond the lobster, it became difficult to tell if she enjoyed going there anymore. Certainly not the plane ride, particularly because I'd always relied on Cheapo to supply our tickets.

But, by 2014, Linda's affect, for the most part, had largely diminished to a quiet inertia, a barely present passivity. With minor exceptions, she put up with us. And, by then, she had begun to lose control of her bladder. I was, and would continue to be right to the end, her primary caregiver. Of course I was. Who could do it better? I couldn't possibly need any help—Linda seemed OK with that, but, then, I didn't really consult her about her preferences for home care. I was the man, mon. Besides, looking back to 1965 and the year of no-holds-barred, full-contact caregiving she had devoted to me, I owed her big-time, didn't I? There was never a question in my mind that I would or could do it as a sixty-eight-year-old guy invading the private recesses of my sweetheart as well as she had for me at a nubile eighteen.

That might have been an acceptable idea at the obvious

start of her mental decline. However, that downhill slide had begun much earlier, as Karen has told me many times since, but I was way too close to be able to chart Linda's regression. No real problems taking over the finances, the house cleaning, the laundry, and the cooking. When Linda's back problems deteriorated to the point that she would need a fusion in June of 2012, I was home to care for her, teaching my summer courses online, and able to transfer her to the Masonic Home in Bloomington for her transitional care and the start of her physical therapy.

When she returned home to our condo in Bloomington—a decidedly '70s building on the first floor with no accessibility features—I began to broach the subject of our moving to one of the many assisted living situations. She would have none of it, though. If her emotional affect was disappearing, it wasn't regarding this subject. She was angrily, aggressively, passionately against it. Part of her resistance, I'm certain, had to do with the comfort and security she felt about clinging to the last major part of her independence. She liked the condo, she said. It was hers.

Gradually her resistance shifted into paranoia. "I'm not going anywhere," she declared. "And you can't make me. I know what you're trying to do—you want to get rid of me, throw me away so I won't burden you anymore." Yikes! Linda would play this song at various decibel levels over the next five years, and I got it. Besides remembering what her mother might have felt when Linda moved Dorothy out of her own home to a strange state and into a succession of nursing homes before she passed in 2010, she was terrified of losing what she had left of herself. No matter how hard I pushed back against that terror, the more she clung to her certainty of it.

But, if anyone reading this might be thinking that I had other options for sharing my care of Linda with other paid caregivers while keeping her in our home as long as I could, I hadn't gotten there yet. I wanted her with me. I was too stubborn to realize that I was probably contributing to her terror.

And, of course, rationalizing to myself that I was helping

her by planning more trips I could brighten her life with. Let's see: between 2014 and 2018, there were three Hawaian adventures. All were difficult for her given the length of the plane flight, but the last one in 2018 to Kauai, which coincided with the installation of a curb-less walk-in shower after I'd installed a pocket door from the bedroom for easier access, occurred in the midst of an historic monsoon that knocked out roads and bridges and dropped another twelve inches of rain after we'd absconded to sunny Maui; a 2015 trip to Nassau and a resort in Cat Island that proved way too strenuous for her; another 2015 trip to an exclusive resort on the Riviera Playa for our fiftieth anniversary during which Linda was treated by the staff like a queen; and a darkly unfortunate trip to Antigua.

And, of course, there was the crazy trip to Sanibel by way of Savannah in winter of 2013, just prior to her second knee replacement, when I stuffed a mattress and bedding into the back of my Subaru Outback, made a recumbent Linda as comfortable as possible given the Siamese kitten she'd be sharing that space with, and drove a car looking for all the world like a hearse with Linda lying in state the entire twenty-five hundred miles down and back. Insanely creative. No seat belt. She did fine with no complaints, regardless of all the folks in passing cars wildly looking and pointing. I still try hard not to think of the danger I exposed her to.

But I've saved the worst, the most torturous, for last. Everything in 2017 and after would be crucial to what would soon become a precipitous decline in her mental acuity and her control over basic physical functions. In the Spring of 2017, we would embark on a three-week tour, beginning in Seattle, moving down old route 1 in California and staying in cottages and bed and breakfast accommodations in Mendocino, Bodega Bay, and Napa, several days in a waterfront hotel in San Francisco, over into Yosemite for a week in a cabin situated at the base of El Capitan, and then back over to the coast to spend time in Big Sur and Carmel before driving to the home of my son and his wife for a visit, after which we'd take our return flight back to

Minneapolis. A great trip for folks in their thirties.

If that journey doesn't sound simple and carefree, it wasn't. Linda and I had looked forward to seeing Yosemite from the beginning of our marriage. And that might have been fine if I hadn't unnecessarily complicated it with the arduous drive (by this time, I should have known that such long road trips were incredibly taxing on her and the challenge of her incontinence), an unreliable rental car, and, once we'd arrived in Yosemite, the realization that Linda had forgotten to pack the narrow and compartmentalized plastic container for her several pills (the most important of which were the Synthroid which served to keep her on an even keel since her thyroid stopped functioning and the medication that stabilized her mental well-being).

Up to this point, Linda was still in charge of that pill box and metering out her daily doses from the day-labeled compartments, which was an act of negligence from the start on my part. It didn't matter that I had asked her before we left home if she had, in fact, put them in her luggage. She was becoming increasingly forgetful by then; Karen and I had remarked on how Linda's mind seemed to operate on a loop. Sometimes, she would repeat what she had already said to us during conversations. Occasionally, those repetitions would multiply. We'd gently tell her that she had already told us what she had repeated, and she'd be surprised that she had done so. Not wanting to throw her into a state of confusion or frustrate her to the point of irritation, we generally ceased reminding her that the story she was telling us was a repetition.

Thus, it availed nothing for me to ask her if she had packed those pills. She truly believed she had; what I didn't do was check what she'd packed to be certain. And there we were, in our little spartan cabin at the base of El Capitan on the eighth day into our trip with seven to go, suddenly aware that Linda was without the things she needed the most. We talked about it and about what we might be able to do. It would have been entirely possible to have Karen locate the container of pills and send them off to us overnight, but I didn't consider that.

Instead, I asked her about the state of her mind, about her level of anxiety without the pills she needed to stabilize her moods. She said that she felt fine and was ready to continue. She sounded and acted calm as well. So, on she went to breakfast and through three more days of being pushed in her wheelchair in every area of the park that I could take her, and a few that I shouldn't have, a successful short stay in the park that she expressed joy in being able to experience.

And on we went to short stays at Big Sur and Carmel before taking the long trek north through Oregon and on to Port Angeles on Washington's northern peninsula close to the Canadian border. It was a taxing ride, made even more so by Linda's near total lack of bladder control. I'd managed that by bringing padded waterproof sheets that I could wash at laundromats along the way, but she had a rather urgent incident along the forested back roads very close to our destination that, because I was unable to find a proper facility for her to use in a timely fashion, upset her greatly. We had burned through many protective undergarments during the trip, but they weren't sufficient to help her during this incident, necessitating a complete change of clothes.

To top off her frustration at being unable to control her own body, Linda was prevented from flying home on our confirmed date when, after she'd boarded and went to use the bathroom, she launched into a loud coughing spell. Linda customarily coughed long and often due to her asthma, with no ill effects, and she was fine as soon as she had accessed her inhaler at her assigned seat. But that wasn't enough for the two cabin attendants who, not swayed by my attempts to convince them that she wasn't ill, insisted that we both deboard the plane. An unexpected inconvenience and source of embarrassment for Linda that delayed our return home by another day.

It's hard to justify any of this to myself. No, impossible. By October of 2017, Karen and I would receive an official professional diagnosis of Linda's gradual loss of mental and physical control. After a series of cognitive tests, it was determined that Linda had developed, by this point and most likely considerably earlier, early onset dementia. The bladder control issues were a direct result of that condition.

But I wasn't through torturing her just yet. There was one final trip I insisted upon taking her on. This one coincided with our annual mini reunion with Pen and Jim in Ogunquit. She eventually would lose her appetite, her neurologist would tell us, but she hadn't yet, and a boatload of lobster rolls, I thought (if I thought at all), might be a temporary restorative. And so it was that I planned a flight to Quebec City, from which we'd begin a journey of eight days around the Gaspe Peninsula, after which we'd wend our way in our rental car across the border and down the coast of Maine.

It's important to note that I sold this trip to Linda as one that she couldn't live without experiencing. The reality was that, as was so often the case in our more than fifty years of marriage, I wanted to take this trip. I'd lusted after it after having been told about its many glories years before by good friends of ours. I convinced myself that I could make this a comfortable trip for Linda and a safe one. Again, I'd pack lots of protective undergarments, lots of padded half sheets to protect her and the beds that we'd be sleeping on in the several B and Bs that I'd booked. But I still hadn't received and absorbed the memo about her inability to bear long road trips without severe discomfort. I compensated by making daily driving distances short and accommodations more frequent. And I capped off my selling job by detailing the visual delights we'd see on our circuit of Gaspe.

As it turned out, I couldn't have been more cruel to her if I'd intended to be. And the cruelty began almost immediately. The second leg of our flight to Canada left us without a great amount of daylight. As we drove scenic 132 toward Rimouski with the broad St. Lawrence River on our left, I knew that we needed to get to our accommodation in Le Bic before dark. And we just made it.

As we pulled up to the quaint and historic Auberge du Mange Grenouille, it looked doable enough for Linda and the little power wheelchair that I had bought her for this trip that she could operate herself on flat paved ground. But our view of things changed abruptly when we were assigned a room at the rear of the building. Getting there necessitated a perilous trip downhill with Linda in her wheelchair and me operating it, across uneven and unstable flagstones and then across wet grass to our room, which required getting her out of the chair and up three stone steps. A nice enough room, if cold because it was late October now and the place was unheated. But the meal we had in the hotel restaurant was excellent.

But later in the night after we'd retired, Linda felt a fierce need to get to the bathroom. In my eager attempt to help her up and through a dark room, I accidentally closed the bathroom door on Linda's index finger. Linda's scream was agonized and electric. Of course, I felt terrible, but the hell with me! This was serious pain that Linda was feeling.

Nothing was broken, but it was clear that one night would be more than enough in this place. I brought her breakfast down to her from the restaurant, but, in doing so, I realized how difficult it was going to be to get Linda up the hill and into the car. It was even worse than the night before because the path up required three stairs down, another three stairs up stone stairs, and then, having to leave the wheelchair, a final eight stairs to traverse before we reached level ground. Pure and exceedingly slow-moving torture.

As I helped her up the final steps and into the car and deposited our very wet laundry in the trunk, I entertained calling it all off, calling ahead and canceling our remaining reservations, and heading back to Quebec City. But no. We soldiered on, with nothing like that first night to reoccur. And, on our final night, several inches of snow had fallen, making Linda's entrance into the car even more treacherous,

The final indignity of this ill-begotten trip occurred on the morning of our departure from Ogunquit. There had been lots of laundry for me to do during our four days at the Beachmere, and I'd earned every bit of it. Now I'd be carrying all our bags while I situated Linda in her power wheelchair so that she could motor up the path and on to the car.

As I rounded the corner laden with luggage, I saw that Linda had collided with a parked pick-up truck. When I got to her, I saw the deep red contusion on her right leg from having impacted the truck's bumper. She was in all kinds of pain—again, nothing broken, but no one could possibly say that I hadn't done everything in my power to hurt her. Awful. Putting a woman with dementia at the controls of a power wheelchair? And what made my guilt even worse was that, almost without fail, Linda didn't strike out at me.

That contusion never went away.

CHAPTER 7

A Fait Accompli: A Visit to Dr. Fuhrman

The concept of fate hasn't played a big part in my view of how individuals are or are not locked in place across the cosmic chess board. It's a mixed bag, it seems to me. I'm not Oedipus nor was Linda, being shoved in apparently prioritized directions amid our own ignorance of who we are toward a deliberate end by decisions we make, the choice of which seems stacked against us. Donald Trump would love such a system, orange ass-hatted blamer of everyone but himself for the regrettable moral and legal fix he's now in—a "rigged system," indeed. But even he in all his Oedipal narcissism would have to admit that, while being overwhelmed by circumstance, we, like Oedipus and Trump, aren't mere puppets ("I'm not a puppet—*you're the puppet*"). We make choices, bad or good, that determine (that's the word!) our paths. Perhaps it's true that our character is our fate rather than the rooting interests of gods or goddesses. We make that fate ourselves until chance steps in to twist it into knots.

There's an exception, though, to the notion that we choose our own fate. Homer couldn't have known it, but it's called genetics. One of the still unresolved influencers of human health and behavior is genetics. Of course, we've been on speaking terms with those double helix-ed strands that make us what we are, determine to what degree we look and think like one parent over another, and prefigure our physiological make-up.

But genetics have been proven to influence our mental make-up, to shape to some unknown degree our tendency toward illnesses of the brain. There's no doubting how Linda's mind and moods had been shaped by her environment—living in close quarters with a crowd of competing, arguing children and adults, skipping back and forth with her mother and brother across the country in search of some domestic definitiveness and stability—and by a small nuclear family led (and I use the word advisedly) by a mom desperately unhappy with herself, her situation, and striking out against constant reminders—her kids—of her restricted lot.

But Linda's mental health was also conditioned by her family. Lots of moving parts here. Of course, there was Dorothy. No yellow brick road for her, to be sure. This woman, if I may be so bold, was without resolve, decisiveness. She was, without Hamlet's immobilizing grief at the loss of his father, his strength of mind, nor the paranoia that comes from living in an environment in which everyone is plotting against him (even Horatio, perhaps), a weak female version of Hamlet.

Whether Dorothy was still in the throes of overwhelming grief at the loss of her husband when I met her, she was certainly playing that role to the hilt. There was passivity in her acting—she'd never be able to take on a role outside of it—but there was also deep depression with an admixture of narcissism, victimization, and self-pity that was real. Living in a fetid swamp of a house ten or so years with no impetus to do anything other than live lethargically and watch TV left quite a visual lesson for her kids. She had gloried in her ability to keep the ever-present middle-aged Donald, who mowed her lawn and made repairs on the house, and the more rarely seen Bob of the phone company on the proverbial hook for many years, never making a commitment nor treating them with respect. But Dorothy was merely one of seven sisters who, like her, suffered from some level of mental dysfunction.

Mostly it was depression, but there was also one suicide and at least three other cases of mental breakdown. Ruthie, Reggie, Edie, Lucy, and Annie all developed varying degrees of dementia. Edie's and Lucy's and Dorothy's were severe. And that's not to mention other women in Linda's vast extended family who suffered mental breakdowns, one in particular, a young woman married to Uncle Dennis (whom Dorothy invited to tow a special interest car I'd sweated over for years out of her backyard while Linda and I were in New Mexico for two years and out to his junkyard) who had experienced repeated breakdowns. The women in her family had seemed especially vulnerable to them and to dementia.

I was considering all these examples of mental illness by January of 2017. Linda's behavior and moods had become increasingly erratic. Besides the occasional loud outbursts of anger, the failures in short-term memory, and her growing habit of talking in a closed loop, she had grown more lethargic. Those crafts she'd taken such pleasure in doing for so many years, and to such great effect, had ceased to interest her. True, she was still making some jewelry and putting it on consignment, but very little.

Besides, she'd lost complete interest in the cabin, in going there, in enduring the long ride; I'd set her up in the old Lazy Boy with the footrest located close to the front wall of glass overlooking the deck and the array of hummingbird feeders that retained a little fascination for her. And there she'd sit for the next two days, moving only to use her walker to get to the bathroom or let me drive her to one of several excellent restaurants for a meal. I was worried about her. This once voluble and happy woman had not only gone quiet, but she'd tuned out. A smile was rare, a laugh was rarer, and full-blown inertia had set in.

But Karen had seen more than I had. When I consulted her about my concerns about mom, she told me that she'd seen what I'd seen for a year or more. What's more, Karen told me that she'd been shocked by what she'd seen in Linda the last time we'd visited her home for dinner. Almost a complete dissociation from environment and others in it. No focus. No interest in anything going on around her. It was almost like Linda was locked inside an impermeable glass case—she could see us if she felt so disposed, but she could rarely hear us, or so it seemed. Karen remembers her seating herself some distance apart from others when we visited her home. It was a rare thing to see her interact, and then mostly with the kids if they'd been successful in engaging her in a game or puzzle.

That's when we started to think about seeking a neuropsychologist for a full diagnosis. It took us a little while to get a referral from those in the know, but, as it turned out, those providing a recommendation consistently delivered the same name—Dr. Fuhrman of Edina. Whether there were a lot of these professionals working in the area or not, it became clear from the start that Dr. Fuhrman's dance card was over-full.

And Linda seemed ok with talking to him and being tested. Or, perhaps, by this point, her apathy had reached the stage where she didn't really care one way or the other. I was grateful not to have become embroiled in another argument with her about the state of her mind—she'd always accuse me of having already pronounced her crazy and that I was just paving the way to her commitment. But this time there was only passive acceptance, not terror. And I remember musing with Karen that, if we were just acting now on what we'd begun to see in her behavior and affect a couple of years earlier, we were indeed attempting to jump on the train after it had left the station and was speeding by us. This would be a crucial marker for what we and she might be able to expect in her coming years, however many of those there might be.

Clearly, Linda had been getting no relief or answers from her primary at a Bloomington clinic who always seemed to listen patiently when we were able to get an appointment to get in to see her but seemed to miss more important signals about Linda than she picked up. She was pleasant enough but ineffectual, and, when it came to carefully observing details in Linda's care like regularly checking her thyroid and the numbers that would tell her that Linda's Synthroid dosage should be adjusted, she dropped the ball. The only good thing she did for us was to recommend Dr. Fuhrman. I was amazed to hear Dr. Fuhrman's voice on the other end of the phone line when I called him in early January. As I was to find out over the next several years, Dr. Fuhrman always answered his own phone!

But, as pleasant and genuine as he came through during that initial discussion, we'd have to wait. Fuhrman's schedule was packed at least until the following October. Sympathizing with me as I described the contours of Linda's mental situation, he suggested that I make an appointment but, if it were possible for us to be ready to respond immediately to a call from him about an unexpected opening because of a cancellation, he would keep me posted. And he was scrupulous about the literal meaning of "immediately": we'd have a half hour to scrape ourselves together and arrive at his office, and no more. So, Linda and I put ourselves on "Fuhrman watch" for the next nine months. Fair enough. He was the best.

Neither Linda nor I was thrilled at the prospect of such a long wait when it seemed that nine months could very well mean the difference between her living or dying. And, of course, Linda wouldn't have been thrilled about anything. She was miles beyond being able to express enthusiasm. By early 2017, Linda was pretty much beyond serious resistance to or even caring about who Karen and I wanted her to go and see. The two of us guessed that dementia would be Fuhrman's diagnosis, but we had no idea what such a diagnosis could mean for Linda's quality of life going forward or even whether that "going forward" would be long or short. We were simply looking for some direction, some sort of confirmation. The falls were occurring more frequently. The protestations and accusations had become commonplace from Linda about the supposed plot I'd hatched for her, how she was convinced I didn't love her anymore and how I'd intended to move her out of the house and away from me so that I could rid myself of the trouble and unpleasantness her inability to care for herself was causing me. Her defenses were set in concrete—there was no other subject that fiercely animated her than that. She'd insisted I'd meant all along to warehouse her as I think she felt she'd done for her mother. Carbon copy. Militant guilt and shame.

Because of my insistence and her apathy, I hadn't entirely given up taking her on trips that I might have done better not taking her on. I suppose it was my way of pushing back on Linda's downward slide away from engagement with life and people. The circuit of her life had largely been reduced to being gently pulled from a dead sleep in late morning into her wheelchair, through the widened opening for a pocket door that I'd installed into the new curb-less roll-in shower that made cleaning Linda up and getting her ready for her day easier. And then it was out into the living room and into her upholstered chair next to the window where I could deliver her poached egg on toast and flip on the TV which would become the focus of the rest of her day.

It was early October when we finally were able to get in to see Dr. Fuhrman. A sudden opening had occurred. It wasn't too much of an imposition to get Linda ready and into the car for the fifteen-minute ride to Fuhrman's office for an 11am meeting in a high-rise building in the middle of Edina. On short notice, Karen was able to meet us there in time for our introduction to Fuhrman, a soft-spoken, kindly man in his mid-sixties. Linda, Fuhrman told us, would be doing a series of cognition and memory tests over the next couple of hours. I'd already explained to Fuhrman what we'd been observing in Linda increasingly over the past year and a half—short-term memory lapses, an intensifying distractedness, an inability to focus, disinterestedness in any of the many activities that had so engaged her over the years, particularly reading. Inertia. Long silences.

There'd also been a steady increase in the number of times she would talk herself into troubling repetitive loops, only several minutes later to pick up the same repetitive loop as if the subject of it were entirely new to her and repeat it all again. Karen kicked in her observation that, in Linda's visits to Karen's home, she would sit apart largely in silence as if in a daze or state of confusion.

Linda had been completely cooperative in responding to Fuhrman's neurological tests, didn't seem bothered at all by them beyond showing some shyness in responding while Karen and I sat in the waiting room. When Fuhrman called us back a week later to share the results of those tests in his office, he confirmed what Karen and I had been seeing. His several-page report indicated some troubling findings: early onset dementia that would gradually worsen, but that we could hope to slow down with the help of medication. Fuhrman hedged on the issue of where Linda stood in terms of the severity of her cognitive decline. While he characterized her mental impairment as "mild" and "not yet widespread or pervasive," her test results pointed to "a general lack of vigilance and concentration." Her short-term memory was "excessively low for her age."

Regardless of her present experience of a mild impairment issue, Fuhrman acknowledged that people, once having begun to decline, continue to do so. The most likely scenario for Linda, he said, would be memory loss "profusion" which "impacts intellect and functioning." Fuhrman backed away from labeling her present state as full-blown dementia but felt confident enough to assert that Linda stood on the edge of early onset dementia. He discussed with Linda, Karen, and me the four drugs that might slow down or stop her mental slippage. There's be no hope for any of them to restore the memory she had already lost nor increase the chance of her holding on to a recollection of names, places, experiences that had just entered her mind. Essentially, her short-term memory was gone. Fuhrman posited that whatever was happening in her brain was too microscopic to show up on brain scans. He seemed quite certain that the years of severe depression Linda continued to experience were not the culprit in her steady mental decline.

Fuhrman encouraged us to try to interest Linda in some

regular physical exercise—more effective, he said, "than mental exercise"—and to work on her diet and nutrition, which, in her present state of obesity, was poor. He prescribed the medication Aricept because it came with no complicating after-effects. It was decided that Linda would confer with her psychologist at the hospital about checking the dosage of her depression medication and replacing Wellbutrin with another depression drug, Zoloft.

So, that's where things sat on October 13 of 2017. Fuhrman had seen what Karen and I had seen: that Linda had become increasingly sedentary and inert. He had noted her long history of major depression and chronic pain, her difficulty in rising from her chair, her instability, and her increasing number of falls. He was able to confirm from his interview of Linda, Karen, and me that she had become "withdrawn and apathetic." In the process, he didn't totally rule out a Lewy body disease, though the chances were remote of her having it given that "stigmata" weren't in evidence but stipulated that it was a possibility that demanded watching. He noted that Linda's mother had fallen victim to memory loss, confusion, and dementia over at least thirty years.

During his examination and testing of Linda, Fuhrman noted several things. First were the tremors in Linda's hands and wrists which had recurred over the previous year and had caused us some dismay. During the tests, Linda had shown consistent anxiety. When she had failed at some points in the memory exercises, that anxiety was coupled with insecurity, Fuhrman had observed. "On the whole," he said, "the test results suggest mild-to-moderate intellectual limitations." Whereas her "recognition memory" tested as "fully intact," her "recent memory" was "markedly reduced," and her ability to "acquir[e] new knowledge and reproduc[e] it after the fact" occurred "with substantial difficulty."

Somewhat disturbing was Linda's performance on tests that measured one's ability to focus and psychomotor abilities: "Ms. Dyer is producing alternating movements with relative difficulty in the left hand but is producing dexterous movements with bilateral difficulty." There was little resemblance between the person who had performed intricate and focused tasks in making her jewelry and pieces of clothing just a few short years previously to this version who had lost the will and ability to move her hands purposively into and through a task.

Of course, we all knew that Linda had become physically limited by her hypothyroidism, asthma, obesity, and chronic kidney disease. But not long-ago Linda had been able to operate efficiently through her many artistic interests. Now those physical abilities were compromised by what we were seeing in these "abnormal" neuropsychological results: "the overall results are compatible with cerebral dysfunction of mild-to-moderate magnitude. The dysfunction is diffuse and bilateral." As Fuhrman concluded, "cognitive impairment is probably the prodrome of a degenerative process. She may be developing an early Alzheimer-like dementia. Because the current deficits in executive attentional abilities and spatial/constructional are greater than usual, she could be followed for a possible element of Lewy body disease."

At the conclusion of his report, Fuhrman closed the book on Linda's prospects for assuming independent control of herself going forward. Others would need to assume full responsibility for administering her many medications, the management of her personal safety, matters related to money and finance, and (although Fuhrman never said so directly) the formal drawing-up of a power of attorney for me and (should I be prevented from executing it) Karen. And, of course, soon indeed, someone and probably others would need to intervene and assist when Linda would fully lose the ability to control her bodily functions.

Meanwhile, Fuhrman recommended that I do what I could and what Linda would allow to get her among people of her age to get her engaged in whatever physical or communicative activity might attract her while educating myself about dementia and Alzheimer's, including area meetings of the local Alzheimer's Association and informational conferences that would occur periodically in the Twin Cities.

Just as Dr. Fuhrman had predicted, things got worse over the next year, necessitating a second visit with him. Given what we'd learned from the first one, both Karen and I became more observant of Linda's behavior and affect. It became clear to us that the apathy, inertia, and prolonged silences were deepening, with the disturbing addition of periods of heightened agitation. So, when we returned with Linda for a second appointment on January 22nd of 2019, we were prepared for an even worse evaluation and prognosis.

But this time Dr. Fuhrman's tests revealed only a "scant change" in Linda's mental decline. He determined that Linda's "memory issues had been confirmed" but that they hadn't really worsened. Certainly, her concentration and focus had "slipped mildly," but Fuhrman was guardedly optimistic about her present mental status, perhaps due to the use of Aricept. Linda's depression had persisted, though improved somewhat with med changes and a significant adjustment in her Synthroid medication after we'd determined that Linda's primary had failed regularly to check its proper levels—perhaps an important contributor to the violent mood swings we'd been seeing.

But, while little had changed for Linda over fifteen months, he warned us to expect greater regression in Linda's formation of new memory and "recent memory retrieval." There would be little we could do going forward besides continuing to supplement her care beyond my caregiving and to take proactive steps to get on waiting lists of several assisted living facilities. We should, he said, expect to have to wait for at least a year for a suitable opening.

Although there would be one more very substantial (and unduly taxing) trip to Maui and Kauai in the spring and a final trip to the Ogunquit seashore in late fall, our lives were about to change radically. By the end of the year, we'd be selling our Bloomington condo—a humble place that Linda felt so secure in—and making a disruptive move into an attractive but (to Linda) strange assisted living unit on the cusp of the Covid pandemic for a year and a half, to be followed by another nomadic turn into another attractive but, for Linda, soon-to-be-frightening new condo environment where she would live her last eight months in varying degrees of confusion, agitation, and terror. From the point of her leaving the Bloomington condo, Linda lived in a constant state of confusion and hallucination about where home was for her and how she could get there.

I recall what Dr. Fuhrman had told us at the end of that second meeting, about how "a mild problem without intervention leads to encroachment into other areas that then slip as well as memory issues increase." That was about to happen in an accelerated way for Linda over a very few short months.

CHAPTER 8

Running Out of Real Estate

For too long, I'd been resisting moving with Linda to a senior facility. I knew how violently opposed to such a move she was, and I knew that I'd have to go too. But I began to look, first surreptitiously, and then, after I'd found a few that I thought were ok and humane, with Karen. She was all for it even if I wasn't. She understood that it was all about safety, along with the delivery of certain attractive (and expensive) amenities. And, boy, were they expensive!

After we'd narrowed the list down to several options with decent food, an open floor plan for the individual apartments, location, and ways for Linda to gain access to other folks she might bond with, we narrowed the list to four: a new one in Minnetonka overlooking 494 and near Ridgedale Mall; the Waters in Edina off Highway 62; Summit Place in Eden Prairie; and Parkshore in St. Louis Park within walking distance of the hospital and a variety of clinics.

It was time to see if I could get a little buy-in from Linda. She was generally disgusted with the whole thing (it was a vast conspiracy being conducted against her) and was fiercely determined to hold on to her little condo with the view out the windows of the forest of sheltering trees and the beautiful garden of flowers across the way outside her friend Nancy's condo. But, to my surprise, she agreed to go on some site visits with me. She never expressed enthusiasm (I think she was beyond such an emotional display), but she clearly appreciated what she was looking at and how being in one of those places might help her in several ways. We toured all manner of living space floor plans, visited the aquatic center at the three places that had them, and were blown away by the costs of living at these places (I was amazed that there was an a la carte price for nearly everything).

So, Linda played it on the down-low, expressing what had become her customary pessimism, but it was clear that she wasn't averse to the idea. Optimistically, she didn't exhibit the kind of resistance that prevented her from letting go of the car's door jambs when I tried to get her to allow me to roll her into the Senior Center in Bloomington because she didn't see herself as old as the seniors inside were. I vividly remember driving into the center's parking lot one sunny Friday, parking the car, getting her wheelchair out of the trunk, and asking her politely to take my hand so that I could help her out of the car. She wouldn't budge. This was quintessential Linda with her heels dug in. I patiently waited for her to change her mind, telling her of all the wonderful classes and activities that I'd seen were occurring inside the door. Nothing. She wouldn't budge. "I'm not going in there, and you can't make me. There's nothing for me in there." In that case, it was her mother all over again—she'd never forgive me for saying that—who didn't want to be classed among them, even though they were so actively engaged in any number of activities that they'd been scheduled to do.

The only real thing that raised flags for her beyond cost (which truly was preposterous) was the relative size of these units. There was no question that we'd need a unit with two bathrooms; I'd had to renovate the ugly basement shower in Bloomington for my exclusive use because so much related to Linda's needs was going on in the primary upstairs one. Space was crucial for me too—I could see that down-sizing was in the offing here—

that was, after all, the point. The basement and two garages had been jammed with cars as well as stuff that I'd need to sort through and get rid of. Lots of trips to ARC and Good Will and, unfortunately, the landfill. Lots of painful decisions to be made. Linda had always been an organized pack rat—all of her craft stuff, which was vast; all her painting supplies and books; tons of clothes, much of which was brand new or hardly used; the endless heavy photo albums that covered every bit of our lives together; a house-full of paintings, some valuable, that we'd collected over the years; tools, both hers and mine; and an endless number of purchases at garage sales.

But the biggest decision we'd have to make—it was so damn final that my internal Hamlet began to rear its ugly head—was to sell the condo, and to do it in a way that would avert being a major imposition on Linda.

Timing was everything. We wouldn't sell it until we were well out of it and in our new place. Once that had occurred and Linda's attention could be drawn to her new digs, getting used to it with her pal and my new co-caregiver Heidi, I could get to what needed to be done to engage a realtor and ready our nearly fifty-year-old condo for sale.

Karen came up huge again. After we'd decided upon Summit Place in nearby Eden Prairie—it would, in fact, be the easiest move—Karen employed a real pro (a friend and neighbor who'd built an astounding reputation among area realtors) who came in, called all the shots about which floor coverings needed to be torn out, which walls needed paper removed and repainting, what furniture needed to be shipped out, and what lighting fixtures needed to be replaced to achieve the minimalist look that she knew would attract buyers.

A host of her people were set to work. I'd already installed a new gas stove a few months back, and a dear ancient friend who'd taught me all the carpentry I'd ever learn had built Linda a kitchen full of beautifully finished natural light aspen cabinets with modern nickel pulls and European sliding drawers only a year before that. My two tiled bath jobs—the neo-angle curbed shower that I'd built downstairs, along with the tile floor for the roll-in shower upstairs that I'd commissioned—gave us a leg up on what would be a very quick sale.

There was just a ton of work hauling furniture and Linda's craft materials to ARC in my F-150, and I'd need to do a lot of running to do business with the retailers who'd be providing materials to transform the look of our old place. Removal of what was essentially fifty-year-old wallpaper was my worst nightmare.

But, when all was said and done, we made an astonishingly large profit on the place after selling it in two days. What a gift, what with everything else we had going on. One of the great gifts beyond selling it was flying my son out to help me for a few days. A brawny and imposing ex-Border Patrol officer now, Chris helped me with the brute work—emptying some of the big stuff from the basement, disposing of the detritus in gigantic bags for the trash man to pick up, and emptying and then cleaning the two garages, a major piece of work.

And then "the move." As near as I can recall, it occurred on January 2nd, and during a very cold weather spike, treacherous for Linda to have to be transported in. I'd never moved like this before. Karen took it all out of my hands and entrusted it to a company of women who, after spending a day carefully labeling and boxing all our belongings, took only another day to move it all to Eden Prairie.

Linda and I had always done it ourselves, renting any equipment and vehicles we needed and enlisting our friends to help us. And no one packed a box or a truck more efficiently or intentionally than Linda. But we couldn't do that anymore. I was game, but my right leg was gimpy from too many strenuous tasks like the roofing I was doing at the cabin.

Karen had successfully arranged the most humane and efficient move I've ever witnessed. My job had been to draw an accurate representation of the space in the new apartment. After I'd gathered the dimensions of each piece of furniture and painting and added each of those personal items to my drawn space of the rooms and walls, I then handed it over to the movers (mostly women who were in the process of meticulously packing everything according to where these packed belongings would eventually be placed or stored). Two days.

When we were finally allowed into our new living space at the end of a long day, it was as if we'd always lived there. All empty boxes had been moved out, every vestige of material that could be associated with the arduous task of moving had been discarded, and all we had to do was thank them, pour a glass of wine, and make dinner. Everything in its place. Karen had facilitated the removal of most of the stress the move would cause Linda. Magic.

But then there was the year and half of living in Eden Prairie. Almost from the start, what seemed like such an open and welcoming place just a short walking distance from a major mall and grocery stores and an animal hospital (I can't forget Raj, our male Siamese; he had his own adjustment to the move), quickly turned into a holding facility.

That's right. Covid. Big time. The news across the country about how nursing homes and assisted living facilities were being ravaged by it worried us, but our experience was different. Yes, Summit Place had active cases of Covid. I'm not sure if people there died of it; we weren't given information on that stuff. But people were sick with it, from the locked wing dedicated to folks with Alzheimer's to the four floors of assisted living and independent living residents like us (we had chosen the independent option because it was the only way we could get an apartment with two bathrooms). But people were—it goes without saying—dying there all the time. That, and the fact that the place was locked down, wouldn't allow direct relatives to enter and visit, and the staff checked my comings and goings like hawks, made this a depressing place.

There was one notable time that I had taken Linda to the cabin just overnight so that I could finish roofing the hardest half of the carriage house. While we were there, Linda sat in her usual place as I prepared the downstairs bedroom for her to sleep in; everything we ate I cooked or brought home from the general store in downtown Cornucopia. But when we returned to Summit Place Senior Campus, we were told that we would be quarantined for the next week because we had stayed overnight near people who could put us and the entire facility in jeopardy.

There were several more of these, mostly involving me, but their decisions about moving around and outside of the community, even if (as was true in our case) we were extremely scrupulous while at the cabin about going to restaurants or food stores, etc., were overly restrictive, isolating (just what Linda did not need), and non-logical. I understand a large corporation wanting to insulate itself from lawsuits and escalating numbers of sick and dead residents at their facilities because most of the facilities like the one that Linda and I found ourselves victimized by were protecting their own asses while locking down, isolating, and increasing the onset of depression among its residents.

And might I say that being in one of these facilities put me on the brink of running out of money, and that's no joke. Lots of people—caregivers like me—were trying to do the best they could (my own deficiencies excepted) to keep their charge happy and healthy while at the same time feeling squeezed by anxiety and depression about paying the bills. Baseline, I paid $4,300 per month just for the pleasure of being in jail, consigned indefinitely to confinement, while an additional $3,000 on average went to the caregiving company I'd contracted with, Eden Pathways, and their minimum wage-driven care workers. That's huge, and at one point I felt it necessary to enlist my MBA degreed son-in-law as well as my investment counsellor in a collaboration to build a plan for amortizing the amount of money we had saved and invested along with the funds we had coming in from my pension and our social security payments—that is, I was building a plan to determine how long I could meet my financial obligations before I couldn't. Bad news.

It was a tough time—I'm certain that Linda was aware that it was. What did it mean for her? Lots of TV. Lots of Hallmark Christmas movies, no matter what season we were enduring. Playing with our Siamese cat Raj (which included my chasing the little guy through the halls and into adjoining apartments when he broke out). Puzzles. My reading *Pride and Prejudice* and other books to her. Meals of questionable quality prepared by me. But our apartment came with the advantage of a big front room with a large picture window that looked out on a lovely open space with a circular seating area, flowers and other plants, and an audibly gurgling large fountain.

Linda and I spent lots of time out there because it was one of the few places we could go. We often sat out there—Linda in her wheelchair which by then had become her permanent seat—and ate our lunches. And, when Linda's favorite caregiver Heidi was on duty, she'd sit out there for hours talking about I don't know what. Kind of like convicted felons permitted to leave their cells and recreate out in the "yard."

Linda had lots of caregivers while there—obviously, Heidi was a popular choice of many patrons of Eden Pathways, so we had to book her when we could. Some of them were irredeemable incompetents, either because they were ill-trained, stupid, lazy (there's a lot of that going on) or made inaccessible by phones stuck in their ears. There's no excuse for this failure—I hadn't hired them to waste my time, avoid communicating with Linda, or show up when they wanted to. I had to repeatedly and frontally call these miscreants out, not always to good effect, and occasionally I had to do the same with the owner of the caregiving company, who is a practicing physician and ought to have known better. I'm not sure how I could have avoided so much of the bad work these caregiving outfits were charging me for without hiring them and finding out the hard way. But I had to start someplace in finding help for me and for Linda.

Suddenly in June nearly a year and a half into our prison sentence, a command decision—who the hell knows if it was the right idea to buy a place and move the hell out of the prison that Summit had become? I guess it was me. Economically, it didn't make sense to stay in such an alienating place. I liked a good number of the people we met and ate dinner with before it wasn't possible to get to know them or anyone else. We were, after all, safe and warm, which had a lot going for it. There was no guarantee I'd be able to find something livable and conveniently located that we could afford if we abandoned Summit.

But there were more important considerations. Increased anxiety for one; that was real for Linda, and she'd shown signs of feeling more of it. But more important still was ensuring Linda's stability. I may not have particularly liked the place we found ourselves in, but Linda was generally happy enough, or as happy as Heidi and Karen and I could guess she was. She wasn't talking much. Not really interested in the practical concerns of the everyday world. And that's when I began to question whether moving her—wherever that move might take us—was the right thing. Better to leave her where she was, now a year and nearly a half of her adjustment to living in a place she never really wanted to move to out of a place she never wanted to leave.

Note that by this time, in the spring of 2021, Linda had pretty much forgotten where she was a year and a half ago. It was all in the moment for her now. Dealing with her needs as they occurred was really all that mattered. By subjecting her to another move, I could very seriously be letting her down, or letting her in for physical and psychological dislocation, maybe even delivering a disabling backsliding blow to her psyche. Besides, forget about the money—it was too late to move her, and for what besides the money? Freedom? Convenience? What's more, I began my search for a new place with a desire to find a single-family home. Crazy. Doing upkeep on a new place while paying close attention to Linda?

It didn't take long to disabuse me of that silly fantasy. It was the height of the real estate boom in Minnesota. The only bargains available were the ones with sliding doors that opened on nothing but two stories of air all the way to the ground; or the single-story with walk-outs with bad kitchens, stairs to descend into the basement (always a basement, finished or not) with endless work to be done for 400K; or homes where my looking stopped at the steep front steps with no railings; or big houses on one level built in the '60s with a few internal short but deal-breaking changes in floor levels.

Others I wanted to look at that seemed potentially workable were sold before I could see them, and there were no handicapped access single-family homes on the market.

Don't ask me why I wanted to buy a detached single-family home other than that we'd been held captive in a place we were merely renting. Besides, the notion of independence in as many things as possible had always been a big thing to me. Again, it was a selfish choice on my part. If I'd been honest with myself and thinking solely about her welfare, I wouldn't have moved her at all. And, in the final analysis, I'm so sad to say, the whole issue of my trying to build a hedge around going broke would be moot, given that Linda had such precious little time to live.

But I found a place, finally realizing that the only real way to get a one-floor handicapped accessible living space (what else? —a flat) would be to buy a condo. And, in no time, I thought I'd found in an online ad just what we both needed, and more. Of course, a mere photo and realtor's hyped description would never convince me that what I was looking at was real or workable. Just look at our place in Bloomington with its narrow door openings, its bowling alley arrangement of rooms opening off a narrow long hall, its crazy two-door openings into the bathroom of 28 inches each, each door opening inward and in opposite directions and guaranteed to create chaos, the ten-stair descent to the landing from which the garage was accessed, never mind the two ninety-degree turns down another two flights of stairs leading to the family room and laundry and storage area. And that leaves out the impossibly narrow thirty-foot walk to reach the car in an overly narrow garage. Linda may have liked our old condo, but it was dangerous for her in so many ways, just as so many of the other condos we'd looked at before we'd bought that one.

But, when I dismissed the realtors' recommendations for more unsuitable houses to look at and their deafness to my pleas to look at condo "flats" that might work for someone who was now totally bound to a wheelchair, I began looking on my own. And, almost immediately, I found what read like just the ticket to fulfill Linda's needs. The thing was located one street off Excelsior, the main thoroughfare in the center of St. Louis Park, overlooking Wolfe Park, a beautiful and expansive rolling recreation area for walkers, joggers, dog tenders, and pickle-ballers with a small lake fed by a bubbling stream and filled with waterfowl. Additionally, bordering the park is an enormous community center and ice rink.

Even more attractive to me were the walkable conveniences: three food stores; a couple of mid-size and attractive strip malls selling everything from hardware and donuts to tennis supplies and paint products; and a full-service pharmacy. At the heart of it all were a wide variety of clinic facilities ranging from emergency and urgent care to more specialized services, all within a short walk, with a large hospital located a mere mile and a half away. And, should I find it necessary to place Linda in a care facility that could deal with residents beset with advancing dementia like Linda, there was one located directly across the park that Linda and I had already visited that we both agreed was well equipped and appropriately welcoming to satisfy Linda's needs.

I sent the ad directly to Karen to see what she thought. The pictures and descriptions were more than intriguing: a long entry hall on hardwood floors that had served as an art gallery for the recently deceased elderly former owner, and, given our expansive native Indian art collection, it could do so again; a very serviceable galley kitchen with upgraded cabinets and food prep surfaces; a ton of large windows admitting lots of brilliant light into a fire-placed living room; a large bedroom with ten-foot ceilings throughout; two huge walk-in closets with deluxe sliding shelves and containers to the ceiling; an additional bedroom for me to use as an office and repository for my long floor-to-ceiling bookcase; two substantial bathrooms with showers (one with a separate deep tub); and an alcove half-way up the entry hall with floor-to-ceiling built-in cabinets and sliding drawers that fit Linda's glass curio cabinet and dining room table and chairs perfectly.

And, in addition to the little twelve-foot long porch off the living room, a large picture window looked out on a large green area with trees and shrubs completely surrounded by the four levels of residences in the building, with a large fountain just outside that window that bubbled and burbled pleasantly, so reminiscent of the big window in our Summit apartment that overlooked a similar fountain and green space. When we engaged Karen's realtor friend who had handled the sale and showing of our Bloomington place to view it, it turned out to be as good as its promotional material. Linda, by this time in her downward mental health curve, was beyond a strong emotional response, but she was impressed.

Perhaps more important as its many attractive features, the entire place was set up with seniors in mind. Much larger than average sized entry doors to the apartment and to every room; much wider than average alleys up the hall, into the kitchen, the very open plan for movement into and out of the living room, down the wide, short hall past the easy-entry two bathrooms, past the second huge walk-in closet and into the expansive and bright well-windowed bedroom. It wasn't going to be cheap, but it was a secure and safe and accessible living space that would be so much more affordable than living at Summit. We were all in.

As I look back on the myriad of mistakes I continued to make in caring for Linda, there's no question that I got it very close to right on this one. All that was needed was for me to contract with a handyman to cut the curb to the shower in the bathroom that Linda would be using to the lowest possible height.

* * *

And then there was Heidi. To return to the caregiver situation that I'd finally begun to address in our last fourteen months at the Bloomington condo, so imperfectly and ignorantly, I had scoured the independent agencies online for leads and then followed up with phone calls. No real luck with any of them, although I remember chatting with a male owner of a small company who talked glowingly about a woman he employed, a senior herself, with the kind of experience and apparent empathic presence that Linda would need. I had gone to the online clearing houses of caregivers who promoted their credentials and experience with photos, availability, specializations, and pay requirements. Dizzying, especially so when I realized it would be necessary to keep track of payroll and tax deduction responsibilities. And there was bonding as well. I had begun calling some of the bigger (maybe corporate) concerns that had a cadre of (let's admit it) cheap help, maybe no more than minimum wage, on offer as well as trained nurses that would come by once a month and do a pro forma assessment of how the "patient" was doing. It was the indefiniteness of it that bothered me. The unknowability of what/whom I would be hiring to attend, hopefully in a vigilant and competent way, the person I loved most in the world.

After having scanned a bunch of free-lancers online and failing to come to grips with the real possibility that some of those resumes I'd been perusing could very well be acts of creative writing (as I'd found in the process of examining job candidates' application materials while chairing personnel committees), I took the easy way out—in late fall of 2018, I called a big caregiving outfit. LifeSpark. I didn't know any better, and, frankly, I didn't know anyone who'd employed caregivers who did.

They had seemed nice enough when we conversed on the phone. I told them precisely what I thought Linda needed; preferably one person who could come in three times each week for four hours each day, with an additional full day and overnight stay on every other Saturday so that I could escape (that's the appropriate word) to the cabin, do some upkeep, work on my old inert vehicles, read a book, and contemplate my navel to get ready for another challenging week just like the last.

And, starting in the winter of 2018-19, it seemed as if it was going to work. I'd told the director of the company on the phone what Linda's health status was, from her two evaluations by Dr. Fuhrman. She was well into dementia now—how far we couldn't know—and she had lapsed into an apathetic state. She needed stimulation. TV couldn't do it. She needed human, caring interaction—someone to talk with her, to engage her in puzzles, board games, jigsaws—but she also needed someone on the alert to respond to her frequent emergency trips to the bathroom; a desire for a drink; a snack; maybe, if I wasn't home or available, a trip to a doctor's appointment or even a movie or a turn in her chair around a mall.

But the major stipulation from me was attending to her safety—being sure to avoid situations that might make her vulnerable to falls—and hygiene: her near total incontinence; the need to keep her clean and dry; the need to do a laundry if I was unable to do it.

We were plagued from the start with folks who might have meant well (in some cases, maybe not) but were disengaged and, either because of a second language problem or timidity, incapable of conversing with Linda. This may be true across the industry, but every person who was dispatched to our home was relatively new to the U.S., new to caregiving, and short on training. From my experience, our situation screams at a tremendous shortfall of dedicated people being paid a decent wage in an area of health care that is exponentially getting worse.

They were mostly nice enough, but flotsam and jetsam. At minimum, place-holders (cigar store Indians dressed in white) for me if I had other out-of-the-house tasks to perform. Otherwise, the rest, as it had always been since all those years before when Linda was getting worse, was on me, and I was fine with that. I'd gotten better at the job, more attentive to details. After the Yosemite debacle, I was the conscientious pill-organizer, dispenser, and purchaser.

As it turned out, the LifeSpark people didn't take Linda anywhere; most of those folks didn't have drivers' licenses, so, as I always had, I got Linda out and to her scheduled appointments. And I even tried valiantly to get Linda to take advantage of yet another of the local Senior Centers in the next city (we could have even played a little bridge together!), but she stubbornly resisted. I'm not sure if it was partly due to the vanity that comes from not being able to acknowledge that you're not as old or as limited as many of those folks who frequented these centers or a kind of false elitism that she was better than those inside.

Meanwhile, my cooking was getting better and more creative. And, once I'd committed to forking out the big money for a roll-in shower and doing a nifty tile job and glass tile border myself, doing a more professional job of bathing Linda.

But soon LifeSpark would seriously drop the ball. It was the beginning of October of 2019, and I needed to drive four hours to the cabin to winterize the place and do a little roofing over the bathroom. I'd need the young woman who came to the house to be with Linda all day Saturday to sleep over in the bedroom in the basement, and she agreed after consulting her boss. The intercom that registered Linda's sleeping sounds and her calls for assistance was set up and turned on, my instructions were typed and printed, pills dispensed (the caregiver could only present those pills to Linda, who would then be required to put them in her mouth), and phone numbers to the cabin and to my daughter's house just a few miles away were placed in the caregiver's hands,

But when I returned home at 8am the following morning, the caregiver was gone, Linda was still in bed, fragrantly marinating, and, after I'd gotten Linda up and showered and given her pills and some breakfast, I was stunned to discover that the wash hadn't been done. We were living in a reality in which the laundry had to be done daily, without fail. And there were yesterday's bed clothes and the wet clothes that Linda had worn the day before in a basket in front of the washer. Unbelievable. Unconscionable. "Care-giving?"

I was furious. And when I sought to communicate my unhappiness at the turn of events that had my caregiver going AWOL—sleeping on the job instead of doing it--I couldn't get through to anyone important beyond the receptionist. I recall that it took me three days to get to talk to the manager of the outfit who had originally come to the house to tell us about her company's "services." I told her what I would repeat in a formal letter I sent to the company—that I was livid at the abandonment of my wife, of her employee's utter failure to do for Linda the most basic but most crucial of tasks before leaving her unattended. Are you kidding me? I informed her that she and her company had broken a contract with me and Linda, that they had placed my wife in charge of an incompetent, and that I'd tell anyone and everyone who asked and didn't about the quality of LifeSpark's services. A week later, a check arrived in the mail paying me for services not rendered, but who cares?

So, this is where Heidi stepped in. I was again forced to find replacements for the dangerous dolts from LifeSpark. No, that's not an accurate moniker to hang on all of them. When I moved Linda to Summit, LifeSpark had an office there as part of their contract to provide support services to Summit residents as well as staff in their locked-door dementia section. But I was sufficiently biased against them to avoid them like the plague.

There was a bit of a lacuna between my shit-canning LifeSpark and hiring a replacement. The same problem—a myriad of self-employed caregivers, but hardly any alternative to a staff-run caregiving agency. But a new one appeared like a toadstool emerging after an overnight rain with the appealing name of Eden Pathways. I knew nothing about them, but I quickly contacted them, indicated what I needed, stipulated imperiously that I didn't want a repeat performance of LifeSpark's incompetencies, and arranged for an interview at our home. In addition to the owner of the agency, a practicing emergency room physician whom I'd soon discover had seriously overextended herself in starting this new enterprise, a lithe young woman in apparently top physical condition with a quick smile and an alert and easy air entered. This was Eden Pathways' most accomplished caregiver, the owner proudly stated.

Speaking confidently and easily, Heidi indicated that she'd had previous experience caring for clients suffering from dementia and Alzheimer's and expressed eagerness to join Linda's team. I was seeing Linda lean into the discussion, smile as I hadn't seen her do much, and show a budding interest in

Heidi. Heidi articulated all the right answers. Her fitness and vitality fooled both of us about her approximate age—later, Linda and I would find, after delving with Heidi into her background, that she'd been married and divorced twice, had a twenty-two-year-old son living with his grandfather in Arizona in addition to a thirteen year-old, had experienced some abuse in one of her marriages, and was most likely into her mid-forties.

We'd also eventually discover that Heidi, besides being a single parent wrangling an occasionally difficult middle-schooler, had recently moved her little family and two Great Danes from Colorado into her mother's house in Eden Prairie with some personally disturbing results. She was an experienced caregiver, but with the prospect of being a great deal more, with her training in physical conditioning. There was a bit of the Hamlet in her, we'd soon discover, given that she was disenchanted with the minimum wage that she'd been receiving in an agency that was understaffed and disorganized but unable to make herself break free by seeking additional training, moving to Arizona to be with her father and son, or establishing herself as an independent caregiver. I hired her on the spot, perhaps the most important health-related decision I'd ever make besides hospice on Linda's behalf.

Her presence paid immediate dividends. Heidi and Linda bonded, plain and simple. I think it was Heidi's breezy, open, and genuine interactive manner that sold Linda. No patronizing an old person weak in body and mind. She was able to meet Linda where she was, to engage her in subjects that interested her like movies and TV programs they liked, places they'd traveled to, family challenges they'd each worked through. Linda was attentive to the stuff that Heidi would easily confide about her son's adjustment problems in school, her mother's erratic behavior that shut her off from her husband and Heidi, their love for big and small animals, working puzzles together and playing cards. Heidi was completely open about having been around the block numerous times, quit school, fled far from home as a teen, and made a number of regrettable personal decisions.

There was no self-pleading in anything she told Linda. She empathized just as much with some of Linda's own concerns about her family members, like the birth of her son's little boy Ronin with an incredibly rare disease called Cockayne Syndrome and the many challenges he and his parents were about to experience. Very quickly, this became a friendship they both invested in. No doubt their deepening interaction contributed to Heidi's ability, whether she intended to or not, to bring Linda out of herself.

Heidi immediately implemented some of her high-grade physical training to help Linda do a little exercising, a little movement in place, getting her daily to cover more ground in her walker. She washed and cut her hair, and they ate lunch together, all amid high-spirited chatting and good humor. When she was called upon to do it, she made Linda more comfortable during showering and toileting than a guy like me could ever hope to. When Linda began to experience fecal incontinence and those incidents occurred in compromising public settings, Heidi had a way of lowering the temperature of the anxiety and embarrassment that Linda felt, and she taught me to do the same when I was faced with addressing those problems, as I would many times.

Totally professional, even keeled from the time that she came on board in late October of 2019 to the bitter end in March of 2022. She was there to care for and distract Linda in that chaotic time of packing up to move from our condo in Bloomington through our near-incarcerated tenure in the "independent living" apartment at Summit. Then throughout our mutual challenges and end-of-life vigil in our new condo in St. Louis Park. She did her best work with the immeasurable help of the wonderful folks from hospice as Linda descended into the depths of Alzheimer's terror.

Heidi, even with a history of chaos in her own life, brought stability to ours. Remarkably, after disdaining the intrusion of an outsider into her home and her own personal space, Linda now welled with the expectation of Heidi's every visit and was discernibly disappointed when Heidi had to cancel because she was ill or had to deal with a behavioral problem at her son's school. "Is Heidi coming today?" Linda would ask me. And, if she was unable to come, "Is she ok? Will she be coming tomorrow?"

I don't want to give the false impression that Heidi had been made the sole administrator of Linda's home health care. First, the very nature of Heidi's status as a part-time caregiver made that impossible. And, because she had responsibility for other clients, we'd need to share her with those others. And that made Linda subject to a great variability of quality in the care she received from others in the Eden Pathways stable.

On an average week, I found myself confronted with a very young woman named Audgenay who didn't know how to do the laundry and who proved it by inadvertently depositing a roll of toilet paper into the machine. It took weeks to rid the clothes and the surrounding environment of the snowy fragments that clung to everything. She didn't mean it; her heart was pure. But she was also shy about informing Linda that it was 10am and she was charged with helping Linda out of bed and into her wheelchair to begin the clean-up and showering and dressing that would need to occur before Audgenay could push her out to the living room to have her breakfast. It was a question of authority, and Audgenay had none. But she meant well and Linda liked her and would listen with great patience as Audgenay would catalog her own difficulties with attending to her new-born infant while dealing with a recalcitrant and sometimes irresponsible partner. She was unaccustomed to making the smallest decisions on her own and would come to me for a careful explanation of how to do the most basic tasks. A wonderful person, but she wasn't ready for prime time.

The third person sharing the care of Linda was another woman who had no business being there, and, after two weeks, I made certain that she wasn't. This young woman's primary responsibility was to schedule the company's caregivers, and a measure of how understaffed this little company was proven by her presence for a couple of shifts each week in our apartment. Always late and highly distracted, she spent the bulk of her time on two cell phones, one of which was dedicated to scheduling and tracking whether those on her schedule were showing up for their shifts. Linda was an apparent after-thought to her, a fact that I made brutally clear one morning when I told her that any essential cell-phone use by her would have to be done outside our residence, that she had entirely shirked the reason why she was in it, and that I didn't want to see her in it ever again.

The message got through, evidently, to the owner of the company who, Heidi told us, had called a meeting of her caregivers to forbid the unwarranted use of cell phones while on the job. As if there should have been a need, given proper training they should have already had, for such a meeting!

The presence of Heidi coincided with a more visible unraveling of Linda's psyche and physical being. Soon after I'd hired Heidi to do three or four shifts each week, including that long Saturday until I relieved her at 6pm, her disorientation increased even as her inertia advanced. Not as much interest in collaborating on jigsaw puzzles; either Heidi did all the work or I finished them. Both Heidi and I took Linda for a wheelchair ride out and around the pretty flowered and treed campus. But she wasn't interested; she was barely there. She'd listen to the stories that Heidi would relate about her son's negative interactions with other kids in school or her struggles to find a new living space for her and her son on marginal finances after having been tossed out by her mom. The silences got longer when Heidi wasn't there. She was clearly losing track of what had happened over the previous few days, never mind the last few minutes, and she began to fall frequently.

It's important to note that none of these falls at home harmed her physically, but they certainly unnerved her and me. Most of them were slow slides from her chair cushion to the oriental rug on the floor. Several falls occurred during getting out of and into bed; her short and heavy little legs with atrophying muscles and the deleterious effects from both knee replacements allowed no flexibility at the knee to enable her to hike herself up and off the mattress easily. And, so, the volunteers from the fire station just a block away through the woods from us in Bloomington had become frequent visitors.

I couldn't do without them until I thought that calling them a few times a week was an imposition and I developed my own sketchy methods for getting her on her feet and into a chair. Crucially, once Linda had slid to the floor, there was no getting her back up on a chair or couch through conventional means—neither attempting to lift her with my own diminishing physical strength or by means of lifting straps, which caused her great pain, worked.

After suffering with Linda the increasing anxiety of these recurring incidents, I recalled how I and some of my erstwhile athletic friends used to practice lifting one or more of us from the ground. The method, very simply, involves using the lifter's body as a fulcrum. That lifter must extend his arms to grasp each of the hands of the person to be lifted who has lain flat with knees bent and each of his feet placed on the feet of the lifter. All that remains is, on the signal of the person on the ground, for the lifter to slowly lean backward, smoothly pulling the hands and arms of the other firmly to a standing position. Almost no effort required. At least that was my experience lifting my Linda, who outweighed me by forty pounds.

Although Linda was initially nervous and skeptical of what we'd be doing, she found that, with her cooperation, we could complete this move in one try. Well, I can argue all I want about my speculation of the safety of this move. With all dangerous impediments removed from the scene, and my certainty, from having tried it, that, should I not be successful in getting Linda off the deck on the first try, the result would be to simply lower her gently to the floor with no injury. And this happened, after which I abandoned my strategy and waited for the firemen.

But I was being stupid. There was risk involved; I was putting undo stress on the arms and legs of an afflicted person with diminishing ability to move or even grasp things. And, in the process, I was introducing a traumatized little person to additional trauma.

But Linda did experience a traumatizing fall that caused her great harm. Before we moved from Bloomington, we'd driven into Minneapolis to see a show at the Orpheum on Hennepin Avenue. We had a wonderful time, but, when the show was over, the lobby was so congested that I knew our best bet was to exit on a side street that would require us to walk about forty yards to get to the crossing of Hennepin and over to the restaurant where we had reservations for a late dinner. When we entered the restaurant, Linda was visibly spent, and, as I held her arm firmly linked in mine and asked a waiter to seat us, I felt Linda, still holding on to my arm, sink to the floor.

It was a polished brick floor that the brow of Linda's face impacted upon. Lots of blood resulting from her glasses breaking above her right eye. Several of us were able to get her up while I called for an ambulance and an EMT. It took longer than it should have, but the professionals arrived and administered aid to Linda, who was found to have a bad cut and a probable concussion—yet another trauma. Because of time and the fact that I had a running car situated outside the restaurant, we eschewed the ambulance and drove directly to an emergency room, where Linda required thirteen stiches to close the wound, got a confirmation on her concussion, and stayed under their watchful eyes until 2am. In a couple of days, Linda looked like she'd received a proper beating, and she had.

The window for taking her out in the public in situations that might be risky for her was almost closed, but I continued thoughtlessly to force it open.

CHAPTER 9

Darkness Falls

I'm going to digress from a discussion of Linda's psychological and physical deterioration briefly, but I hope to justify it momentarily.

In 1961, a phenomenon in publishing occurred. A little-known writer named Joseph Heller published *Catch-22*. It was not an immediate hit as a hard-cover, but it sold many millions once it was released in paper-back and its popularity continues to this date even after having been banned many times. Its special fiftieth edition re-release with illustrations put it right back on the best seller lists. One of the greatest and blackest satires of all time, it depicts an America enmeshed in World War II, but not in an heroic or patriotic way. To the contrary, America's generals of Heller's book were craven, grasping charlatans seeking positive personal press while running the war like a capitalistic enterprise. The person who appears to have been running America's war effort is Milo Minderbinder, a first lieutenant mess officer who runs a world-wide operation of buying and selling goods and services on the black market—even military armaments, signing contracts with the Germans that included the bombing of

America's bases and killing American soldiers—for a profit. Everyone in the armed services is understood to be a shareholder (and, by extension, all of us who have bought into the greed-driven American free enterprise system that Heller is pillorying). When he pilfers CO_2 cartridges from flotation devices, he leaves paper shares in their place.

I loved teaching this book. I made many a class read and write about it, long after the book had ceased to be a best-seller. I'd taught it so many times that I nearly had the whole of it committed to memory. It had spoken loudly to me of the pursuit of profit at any cost, of substituting business for morality, of making false gods of those who best succeeded at it, and of criminally indicting the "Christian" god of giving birth to a hot mess and mindlessly abandoning it.

The novel tells the story of a bombardier named Yossarian who, along with his and others' flight crews, was made to fly an ever-escalating number of missions over Italy. The mess officer in his squadron, Milo Minderbinder, becomes a megalomaniac who forms M&M Enterprises to buy up the entire Egyptian cotton crop and, when he can't sell it, coats it with chocolate and has it served in the mess hall. Yossarian is the book's anti-hero who, when the young tail gunner Snowden is killed by enemy flak and spills his guts all over Yossarian's uniform, discards it after his plane safely lands and spends the rest of the war naked, often sitting in a tree as a protest against Snowden's death.

The incident in the plane during the bombing mission over Avignon during which Snowden is killed occurs very late in the book but has happened much earlier in the actual chronology of the plot; it is the book's emotional and moral center, and its impact upon Snowden is prefigured many times during the novel. Only a few pages before the end, Yossarian walks to the back of the plane and sees that the youthful Snowden has been hit. He attends to what he believes is a wound in Snowden's thigh and reaches for the medical kit. After wrapping Snowden's thigh in bandages, he looks inside the kit for the morphine that will reduce the bleeding and address the pain, but, in its place, he finds only a paper share with M&M enterprises printed on it and some packets of sulfanilimide.

Suddenly, Yossarian senses that he has overlooked a more serious injury from the gathering pool of blood staining Snowden's flak suit. As he carefully unzips the suit, he sees the gaping hole in the back of it that had shredded Snowden's internal organs and causes them, including the stewed tomatoes he'd had for lunch, to spill out on Yossarian and the deck of the plane. Through all of it, Snowden weakly whispers repeatedly "I'm cold…I'm cold." And, as Yossarian's narcissistic confidence that he could help Snowden evaporates into a full awareness of his own helplessness in the face of death and a contemptible, incompetent god, Heller's narrator characterizes the reality of the scene:

> Yossarian was cold, too, and shivering uncontrollably. He felt goose pimples clacking all over him as he gazed down despondently at the grim secret Snowden had spilled all over the messy floor. It was easy to read the message in his entrails. Man was matter, that was Snowden's secret. Drop him out a window and he'll fall. Set fire to him and he'll burn. Bury him and he'll rot, like other kinds of garbage. The spirit gone, man is garbage. That was Snowden's secret. Ripeness was all. 'I'm cold,' Snowden said. 'I'm cold.' 'There, there,' said Yossarian.[3]

Narcissism comes in a variety of flavors, I've found. There's the orange-haired, man-tanned loutish and loud version that sees himself as the unquestioned center of the universe, untethered from empathy for others and seeing no value in anyone but himself. But there's another kind—one represented by a desire to hide from others, to seek anonymity in a cloak of false self-sufficiency emblematized by talking to oneself rather than with others because one's own voice provides the best companion, along with a belief that he needs to be the organizer

---

[3] Joseph Heller, *Catch-22* (New York: Simon and Schuster, 1961), 429-30.

and controller of his own small world. Yossarian could provide an example of the latter type. But I'm thinking that, at one time or another in our lives, most of us find in ourselves at least a little of Yossarian's alienated narcissism. That type of narcissism fits me like a glove and resides at the heart of so many of the mistakes I've made regarding Linda.

Linda and I had barely moved into our new condo in St. Louis Park—it had hardly been a month—in such a beautifully landscaped environment when more problems with Linda's health arose. It was the end of July of 2021 when my son Chris, his wife Geana who was a registered nurse, and their star-crossed baby boy Ronin arrived for a visit. It was still Covid time, and we needed to take care about interacting, particularly in a restaurant setting, and be equipped with masks. Strange times, at the height of the pandemic, which posed major threats to both Linda and little Ronin.

After the dinner in Edina—with Chris and Geana; Hunter and Karen; Linda and me—Geana texted to Karen about her concern over Linda's skin pallor, her visible mental confusion. Geana and all of us knew what a wonderful once-in-a-lifetime meeting with her little grandson this had been for Linda, so long in the waiting, and perhaps her only chance. But Geana's immediate concern was for what she was observing in Linda, about the tremors in her arms and hands, her wandering focus, and how what she was seeing pointed toward Linda's oxygen becoming dangerously low. She recommended to Karen that I take her to the emergency room as soon as possible.

Next day I took her to urgent care, but to no avail after waiting with her for three and a half hours except for a recommendation to take her to the emergency room. It was, as I recall, a Saturday night, prime time for all the crazies and drunks and jacked-up nimrods either being held by the cops or looking for a little temporary shelter. Mobbed and noisy. We took a number, sat down, and waited.

After a nearly four-hour wait amid the unwanted entertainment of belligerent and profane men, some in cuffs, arguing with nurses and hospital guards (my son now serves as one in a similarly chaotic emergency room in Plattsburgh, New York), Linda was finally called to be examined. Because it was now after 1am, not much could be done but to take her vitals. But, since her oxygen level was determined to be borderline, her attending doctor ordered that she be admitted for observation for a few days. However, since this was still deepest, darkest Covid time, every room was filled, and Linda spent her first night sleeping in an emergency room examining area.

After she'd been moved to a hospital room, the staff of doctors and nurses went over her thoroughly. Although they found little that we didn't already know, they confirmed the tremors, the instability, the dizziness, disorientation, the overwhelming physical weakness, and a troubling oxygen deficit.

Additionally, though, their diagnosis included vertigo, which they traced to a vestibular disorder. It's impossible to know how long she'd been experiencing this condition, which relates to the three stones in her inner ears which had fallen out of their separate seats. Imagine a small hand-held plastic rectangular game that you might have played with as a kid. Inside that container was a small flat field with three little depressions and three little silver balls which you must try to jiggle into those little depressions all at the same time. And that was what was going on in Linda's inner ears. Those little rocks had been dislodged from their containers, causing extreme disorientation—vertigo. It was up to the folks in physical therapy to engage Linda in a battery of exercises which she'd have to keep practicing to re-seat those stones.

Who knows how Linda had developed this condition. Could it have been triggered by a fall? Absolutely. But not necessarily. Any number of things could have initiated it, including medications she'd been taking, an infection (not particularly likely), or some sort of brain trauma beyond simply falling—and she'd been piling up those traumas, not just physical ones, since she was a child.

At the end of three days, the vestibular problems persisted

(so much like the disorientation Heidi, Karen, and I had seen ratcheting up in Linda for years), and she was sent several miles away by ambulance to a transitional facility to continue working on the vertigo issue and her diminishing strength. She absolutely hated the place and badgered me each of the seven days she was kept there under observation to get her out and home, the designation of which must have further confused her because she'd barely lived there. She particularly disliked the use of the transfer machine that lifted her out of her hospital bed and into her wheelchair at the beginning and end of each day and being ferried to and from her two-a-day physical therapy sessions three times during that week. Even though Linda's taste buds had become immobilized from everything except the chocolate milk and cannoli I'd deliver her each day, this was a woman who had known how to cook and bake well. And, when she reviewed the house food as terrible, I accepted it as fact.

Linda's time at the transitional facility was not entirely ill-spent. The quality of the work and personality of PT therapists there was highly variable, but Linda was lucky to have been assigned to a young Russian émigré who worked patiently with her and introduced several new exercises into her daily routine that were designed to strengthen her legs. Also, the facility was located next to a vast expanse of rolling land, some of which was used for high school football practice. But the rest of it was for public use, with a paved trail wending through and around it and a little lake with benches. Linda and I spent a lot of time wheeling through this beautiful area filled with people getting their steps in and exercising their dogs.

But, after eight days, Linda was done. Even though the folks there wanted to keep her for several more days to work on her strength and balance, she'd have none of it. We didn't wait for the nurse to dress and clean her up; Linda pressed me to do the preparations, and we left without fanfare.

When we finally returned to our new condo, Heidi was able to join us there and continue her service to Linda, and they were having a gay old time, with Heidi steering Linda's chair around the park to their penultimate place on a bench by the little pond to feed the crowd of ducks. I don't think Linda particularly liked being at the new place or, perhaps more accurately, she may have reached a point beyond caring where she was. Apathy had nearly fully set in. I'd been able to come to a small accommodation with the physician/owner of Heidi's caregiving outfit that made Heidi our exclusive caregiver three shifts each week. From Friday until Monday, though, Linda was in my increasingly vigilant care since I was beginning to see where this was surely going.

I hadn't been quite honest with myself about how Linda was running out of time. We hadn't gotten any clear understanding from Dr. Fuhrman or the other neurologist Linda had been seeing at the hospital about how quickly she had been declining or whether the medication was helping to abate that decline. In fact, I never really dwelt on the question of her imminent death. Based on what we had or hadn't been told, I blithely invested in the fiction that Linda would continue in her current state indefinitely as my passive but much-loved companion.

After all, look at the history of longevity in her mom's family. Dorothy had died at ninety, her oldest sister at ninety-five, one at ninety-eight, and three of her other sisters somewhere in their nineties. Dorothy was the youngest to die, I believed, because she hadn't at all taken care of herself. I was still convinced—and I told her nearly every other day—that Linda would outlive me by twenty-years. And I believed, too, that her relationship with Heidi would buoy her, keep her mildly interested in her ever-shrinking world, and give her reason to wake up every morning, no matter how late in the morning it was.

Because that's the way things had been drifting for a long while now—later and later wake-ups, increasingly more difficulty in convincing her that she should leave her bed, no matter how sodden with urine it had become, to move with my help and her walker or the wheelchair to engage in the ever-more difficult processes of showering and dressing. Her will to move was evaporating with every passing day, and, furthermore, it was becoming riskier for her to move at all. There were no more supervised walks with her walker from bedroom to bathroom or from living room to kitchen and back. Too dangerous. Linda's stability, her ability to stand with back straight and eyes looking forward, was nearly gone.

During Linda's hospitalization, I realized that something needed to be done with the curb into the shower she'd be using. Any curb, however small, into the shower, was beyond Linda's ability to negotiate. And that was the one area in our new place that hadn't been made handicapped-accessible. It was explained to me by a contractor whom I'd sought a quote from that, because it was impossible to know what kind of substructure our two shower pans were built over and because our building association had strict rules about getting approval for doing something of the sort I had in mind (that substructure was most likely steel, a deal-breaker in removing the entire six-inch curb), a totally roll-in shower was out of the question.

So, I devised a system by which the six-inch curb was cut a foot from each end and narrowed to three inches, with a smooth cap epoxied over it to ensure its safety and permanence. Because the door to the bathroom Linda would be using was opposite the entry door to the laundry, and because those very large and heavy wood doors often extended fully across the width of the hall and collided with each other, interfering with anyone who desired entrance into the bathroom, I switched the hinges to the opposite side of the bathroom door and reinstalled the huge and heavy solid wood thirty-six-inch door, after which I purchased a clever magnet on the wall trim to keep that door from swinging while Linda was being moved into and out of the bathroom. What's more, I had a veritable battalion of grab bars installed in the shower area, a shower seat inserted, along with a nifty heavy-duty retractable bar next to the toilet.

Even so, Linda was an absolute liability in there. Her legs would no longer help her to raise herself from the toilet. The walk from the toilet to the shower, a mere six feet, proved almost impossible for Linda to do on her own, even given the three-foot sink area that would provide support for her.

It soon became necessary to wheel Linda from bed to toilet before helping her use her walker to step in to her shower and then shift into the shower chair. A major and complex operation requiring many adjustments that needed to occur several times each day. But she begrudgingly complied.

From the time that we got home from the transitional facility until hospice would appear on the scene, Linda declined rapidly. It wasn't all over for her yet in terms of getting out into the fresh air a couple of times each week. By the third week in September, however, the weather was turning cold. It was a job getting Linda's winter coat, gloves, and her favorite purple hat on along with a wool blanket to keep her warm.

Heidi and Linda would make a circuit, first up our little street to the corner where Heidi could stop for her large caramel macchiato and a sweet nosh for Linda and then down the hill into Wolfe Park, out and around the wooded edge of the wind-protected expanse, over to sit by the ducks to make sounds that attracted them, then around and down toward the rear entrance of Parkshore Senior Living, a place that we had visited before we moved to Summit. Interestingly, we liked it as much as the place we ultimately chose, even though I got a better and friendlier vibe from it. I'd put down a $500 deposit on it, and, after we'd chosen Summit, I let it ride just in case we needed it and insured that we'd be at the top of their list if we did.

Turning right on the path in front of Parkshore, Heidi would wheel Linda past the pock-pocking of the oldsters playing on the pickleball courts to the bridge over the little stream that fed the duck pond and then around and back up the steep hill to the entrance to the Grand Way condos.

This bracing walk generally consumed a good hour of Linda's afternoon when she'd consent to take it. What a wonderful sense-stimulating activity for her! But, by the beginning of October, even that experience became too much. We'd already cancelled our annual journey to coastal Maine for our reunion with Pen and Jim and all the lobsters within our reach. Even Linda grieved over that loss though it was clearly becoming difficult for her to summon enthusiasm for anything. Though she couldn't remember our last trip to Ogunquit, I vividly recalled our flight back and the contained fecal incident she was able to endure until our plane landed in Minneapolis.

Toward the end of the month after enjoying a one-woman show at the Guthrie entitled "What the Constitution Means to Me," I was struck between my narcissistic eyes with the reality of just how little control over the movement of her arms and legs she had when I attempted to help her into the front seat of our car out on the street after the show. I've agonized over the discomfort I caused her on our ride home. This would be the final time that Linda would leave the house to do the very last of the things that she loved.

She had almost entirely lost her ability to support herself with her legs, to exit her bed unaided, to move by herself from chair to toilet. Fecal incidents became regularized, and I can't imagine what that might have done to whatever remained of her self-awareness. No more games, as she was brought to and seated on the couch situated in front of the enormous window that gave way to the view of the now unflowered pergola and waterless fountain. No interest in anything except for an occasional movie on Hulu or Netflix or the streaming of the entire series of "Doc Martin" on the gigantic TV I'd bought for her mounted over the fireplace.

That was all the interest she could muster until the darkness of early winter and standard time introduced Linda, Heidi, and me to the next unforeseen stage of her awful journey.

Heidi was by then on a four-day schedule with us. Since she lost a client in an advanced stage of dementia to an assisted living facility nearby, she now had Fridays available, and I snapped her up. Things were getting arduous, even frightening, and even I knew that having a skilled caregiver for four days each week could only be good. But I took her on privately for that extra day, paying her "under the hat" out of pocket because I could pay her what she was worth rather than the paltry sum her boss was paying her. I'd need all her knowledge and experience, I knew, to learn and implement all of the lifting strategies as well as the essential complex operation of changing the entire bed with her in it.

We would put Linda to bed as early as she'd let us, which usually meant between 7 and 7:30. But, in order to do so, we'd need to carefully work the transfer of Linda from the couch into the wheelchair and then into the bathroom so that she could use the toilet and we could clean her up (shower her if necessary) and dress her for bed.

But then it happened. I didn't know what was happening, but Heidi did. Night terrors. When the sun went down, she explained, the terrors would most likely begin. Awful. Nothing like it. I can't imagine what Linda was seeing in her mind's eye that precipitated such powerful resistance to moving her into her wheelchair. A chaotic thrashing and pushing against the person who had become her best friend, never mind me. It would take the two of us, slowly and with as much gentle reassurance as we could muster, to lift and manipulate her into the chair. It was an exhausting expense of effort for both of us as well as Linda. That determined resistance against neither we nor she knew what drained her into a quivering lump.

But that was just the beginning: whatever it was that terrified her about entering the bathroom, it was real to her. The pushing and writhing that she exerted to prevent us from removing her clothes and sitting her on the toilet was something that I'd only seen in "One Flew over the Cuckoo's Nest" or in a documentary on Bridgewater State Hospital called "Titicutt Follies" many years before. And then the full-throated screaming ensued. Sometimes at the end of Heidi's shifts, she'd stay late until a completely wasted Linda had been deposited in her bed, her pills had been dispensed, and she'd lapsed into unconsciousness.

This, indeed, was a new phase. I hadn't ever been told about how the end of dementia can give way seamlessly to

Alzheimer's (actually, just a more specialized, evil adjunct to dementia), nor, even, how to distinguish one from the other. I'm not sure anyone can with precision or guesswork. Eventually, I'd be told by a hospice manager who came to the house to evaluate Linda that she had crossed over to Alzheimer's. And that is what was entered on her death certificate. But we had a distance to travel before we got there.

Meanwhile, when, almost literally, it was "a quarter to three and there's no one in the place except her and me," Linda would snap me bolt-upright in my bed (I had been sleeping in the adjoining room for more than a month now) with the loudest screams I'd ever heard. She'd always talk through her breathless screaming and inconsolable sobbing to the point of hyperventilation with repetitive phrases like "help me!" or "stop them" or "make it go away." In the dark, it was even more terrifying, and I wanted to avoid any shock that might come from suddenly turning on the lights. Although I was embracing her and rubbing her hands and face while I desperately tried to talk her down, she may not have been able to feel or hear me for the duration of the terrors.

When they stopped, and they eventually did, I sat stunned in the stillness, occasionally wondering if those residing in the apartments adjoining ours and across the hall could hear the screaming and if they were on the phone to the police to report a murder in progress. But it became clear that our apartment was built like a castle keep. Oh, the marvels of sound proofing.

So that tiny bedroom next to hers containing a little twin bed became my outpost, with my ear to the wall to listen to Linda's pattern of breathing to try to anticipate when the next violent outburst would come. The last week of October into the second week of December was a period filled with these heart-rending explosions. Heidi and I both knew what made them come but knew there was no way to avert them.

I recall one particularly nasty event involving the three of us that began on the couch and ended with Linda tearing away from our grasp and nearly falling to the floor. Linda was so loudly and emphatically pushing back at Heidi's attempts to reassure her that we only wanted to help her. I was shocked by Linda's rejection of Heidi's calming words; this was, after all, a person who knew what she was doing, had worked to overcome what were apparently hallucinations many times before and who had become Linda's trusted friend and companion. That was all out the window at this moment as Linda pushed back so hard against Heidi, as strong as Heidi was, that it even caused her to doubt her ability to control her.

During those times, we simply didn't exist for Linda; she had erased us with her rapid-fire "no-no-no." After we'd finally succeeded in settling her into her bed, Heidi and I left her room and, for a few long minutes, looked at each other without speaking. We had no real way of knowing then, but Linda had drawn us with her into her entrance into Alzheimer's.

The night terrors could and would occur daily for Linda anywhere between sunset and pre-dawn, and multiple times through the night, although they usually happened just once each night, probably because of the mental exhaustion each event cost her. And, from this point, whenever Heidi arrived for her next shift, she'd ask me how the night had gone. Pretty much always the same—a largely sleepless night dotted with loud calls of "Bill! Bill! Help me!" and the sudden eruptions of mostly incoherent screams and sobbing. Neither Heidi, with all her experience, nor I had an answer to what was unfolding, short of sitting with her through the terrors and making sure that I was giving her all her medications.

There was no taking her out of the house to see a doctor. And, for reasons I can't plumb, her primary in Bloomington, in a note entered on Linda's MyChart, seemed to cut herself adrift from any further consultations about Linda's mental deterioration. To provide myself some temporary distance from the darkness that had become our home, I customarily left Linda in Heidi's care while I took an hour's walk through the park, past the hockey rink, and down Parkshore Drive to Lund's grocery store to pick up a few items like cannoli and chocolate milk and soups I knew she'd like—she was barely eating and she had clearly lost considerable body mass.

But this time I stopped when I reached Parkshore Senior Living to investigate whether it might be in Linda's best interest to enter their facility. I felt that I'd reached the end of my rope, that insisting upon keeping Linda at home might be doing more harm than good. Besides, I'd continue to be just minutes away in the condo above the park, and I'd be prepared to visit her multiple times each day and, in ways they'd allow, be able to contribute to her care.

I made an appointment to meet the director of Parkshore the following week, at which time she indicated that she'd try to bring with her a nurse who was expert in addressing the needs of dementia and Alzheimer's patients. When the meeting began, the director apologized that the nurse in question might not be able to join us, but, a half hour into our discussion, the nurse appeared. She was sympathetic to Linda's and my predicament, but pessimistic about how Parkshore, given my explanation of Linda's physical and mental state, could help her. I was doing the right thing, she said, by keeping her at home with a regular caregiver and companion that she loved in a familiar environment where she generally felt safe and secure. Parkshore, she said, would effectively uproot her from all that once again and would probably be able to do little more than act as caretaker.

Also, I'd be doing a disservice to myself in the process; first, it would be crazy to consider replicating at Parkshore what I was already doing too much of at home—insisting upon being present and trying to do the work of caregiver there—and, secondly, I'd be prohibited by law, and rightly so, from trying to do Parkshore's work for them. Of course. Dope-slap.

And that's when she incidentally admitted hospice into the conversation. "Have you contacted hospice?" she asked. I was taken a-back. "I have always understood hospice to be the subject of last resort," I said. "That's where people are sent who are adjudged terminal and where they spend their final two or so weeks, right? And Linda isn't close to being there yet." Well, mostly, she said. But not always. "It depends," she said. "I've known cases in which people spend up to a year in hospice. And end-of-life determinations can be a slippery slope. If the hospice community decides that your death isn't imminent, but you've decided on your own, given your doctor's prognosis, to end all medical interventions into your situation and spend whatever time you might have left in a hospice environment, you could very well qualify."

Because I wasn't equipped back then with knowledge of former President Carter's independent decision, at 99, to do just that and successfully seek admission to hospice, as did Rosalind, so that they could be together to the end, I couldn't fully appreciate what she was telling me. And I was way too invested in my own and Linda's problem to appreciate her advice. But, when she suggested I contact the hospice unit at the hospital for a consult, I agreed to investigate.

But with mixed results. When I returned home, I informed Heidi what I'd been told and immediately placed a call. When I got the hospice director on the line and explained Linda's situation to her, her response was discouraging. "It doesn't sound, based on how you've described her dementia, that she could possibly qualify. You've related two instances of testing and diagnosis by Dr. Fuhrman for early onset dementia over the last three years. It would seem that more time and additional testing would need to transpire before we could evaluate her."

Clearly, she couldn't see what I'd been seeing. I guess I wasn't surprised; her response coincided with my initial understanding of how hospice works that I related to Parkshore's nurse. But, before I ended the call, I was able to get the hospice director to agree to do an on-site observation and evaluation of Linda just for our own information.

A few days later in mid-afternoon on the thirteenth of December the hospice director and a member of her team arrived. Heidi had already washed and dressed Linda, and we both explained to her that visitors would be arriving soon representing the hospice organization. This was going to be merely an informational visit, I told Linda, an opportunity to get independent professional eyes to evaluate how she was doing, not too different at all from the occasional home visits from Heidi's physician/boss or the occupational, physical, and memory therapists who still came to work with Linda: "Nothing to worry about, sweetheart. You're not going anywhere. We don't want to be talking about you without you in the room and able to speak for yourself if you wish."

And there she was on the couch in front of that brilliant window, sitting next to Heidi, when I led the hospice people up our long entry hall covered with large works of native American art that Linda and I had collected over the years and into the living room. I drew two chairs near the middle of the room in front of the large glass table directly across from Linda while I sat on a hassock next to the hospice director.

My eyes were fixed on Linda the entire time she was explaining what hospice was and how it worked. There was absolutely no affect in Linda's attitude, but it was clear to me that she was there, listening to all that was being said about the organization and then, very pointedly, about her. She was staring at me, not aggressively or inquiringly but passively as I forthrightly described what I understood to be Linda's career of dementia. A diminishing lack of focus. An increase in disorientation and physical instability. Living in a state of inertia, suspended animation. A withdrawal from all previous interests in her heretofore active life. A near flat-lined apathy. The long silences. The loss of control of her bodily functions. Her increased vulnerability to falls. And, then, finally, the unnerving night terrors that were occurring with disturbing regularity.

The meeting went on, with important feedback from Heidi but not one word from Linda who had barely moved from her slumped position, for little more than half an hour. Again, Linda fully saw me. It was almost as if she was looking right through me. At that point, the hospice director asked me what I understood Linda's wish to be going forward. "To continue to live in her own home with those who loved her for as long as it was physically possible," I said with eyes locked on Linda's. Rising from her chair, the hospice director instructed her associate to immediately call the hospital and have shipped to our home a hospital bed. I was blown away. "Do you mean that Linda will be entering hospice care?" I stammered, to which she responded, "Immediately. In-home. We want to do everything we can to make her comfortable in the time she has left."

But I needed clarity here. What did she mean by "time she had left?" I'd never had any definite sense of that. I was still looking directly at Linda when I asked. Not a glimmer of a reaction when I was told "up to six months." Wow. I didn't know how to read Linda. Probably nothing to read. Was she relieved to hear that she'd be nearing the end of her struggles?

One thing seemed certain: per the hospice director's instructions, Linda would be going to bed and never getting out of it. No more painful and terrifying trips to the bathroom—Heidi and I would take care of all of that. And, emphatically, no more pills of the sort that she'd been taking. All prescriptions would be cancelled because there'd be no need to continue them if, by the very meaning of hospice, Linda would be removed from all medical interventions. In a way, she'd be free. Hospice would prescribe whatever palliatives—either narcotic, which I hoped to minimize unless essential, or otherwise—were necessary to end the night terrors (yes—there were medications that would do that job) and alleviate her pain.

It was going to be all about making and keeping her comfortable right to the end. And that meant access to the full panoply of hospice services: baths and hair-washings twice each week; a music therapy person who'd be coming in at least once each week with her keyboard and vocal abilities to take Linda's requests and engage us in song; pastoral care for both Linda and me when and if we needed it; a cadre of nurses trained to deal with Linda's end-of-life needs 24/7; a doctor in place to oversee every aspect of Linda's care; and a social worker who would be prepared to help me know what I needed to know going forward toward the inevitable.

By six o'clock, the bed had arrived, was set up, and Linda was in it. And, in another fifteen hours, after I'd stowed our queen-sized bed frame and mattress in the enormous storage closet in the front hall and festooned Linda's new bedroom walls with strings of Christmas lights and colorful ornaments, many of which Linda had collected at end-of-season sales years before, the first of an impressive number of nurses, Christine, arrived to carefully and empathetically meet and oversee Linda's every need.

Christine was very young, enthusiastic, and deferential toward Linda and me. She meant for all the world to remove the pressure of what lay ahead for Linda. She took great pains to explain the drugs I'd need to dispense from syringes under Linda's tongue to ease the pain, first one syringe of haldol to be given at the first sign of pain and then additional doses as needed. Only after the administering of haldol failed would I need to introduce the morphine-based syringes, and only after a short time for observation had elapsed.

Christine would visit us nearly every day to check on Linda's status and level of pain, checking her vitals and carefully unpacking our evaluation of how the previous night had gone. Christine would make sure that the supplies of chucks (the absorbent half-sheets under Linda that would contain any fecal material and liquid waste that Linda would pass), swabs, cue tips, cleaning materials, skin creams, and pain-killing drugs would be ordered and delivered immediately as needed. She indicated that the two cotton half-sheets that I'd been placing under Linda would still be useful, only now they'd be situated underneath the chucks.

She and Heidi gave me a short lesson on how to change those chucks by gently rolling Linda, as if gimballed to a hammock below deck, from one side to the other as I tightly rolled the soiled chuck, pushed the new chuck underneath it, and, after one more roll of Linda to the opposite side, pulled out the dirty laundry at the same time as I pulled and smoothed the clean one under her. Finally, while apologizing for the pain that it would continue to cause Linda, she inserted the vaginal catheter that would prove to cause almost as many problems as it was meant to alleviate.

All of that occurred at the end of a long but hopeful night into day opening on Tuesday, December 14th. Heidi and I looked at Linda, now quiet again after submitting to a syringe of haldol, and breathed a long sigh of relief. We had some answers now. Linda had graduated into Alzheimer's. The biological clock was loudly ticking with the imminence of her end. And we now knew that our teamwork going forward would be more important than it had ever been. Our jobs were going to be every bit as crucial as what the hospice team would do for us. We were more than custodians over Linda; we'd be delivering important parts of her care with vigilance, and the hospice team would be relying on the accuracy of our reporting what we did, why and when we did it, and how Linda responded to it so that they could pick up the ball and carry it forward the next morning. I don't think either of us had a hint of how tough our jobs were going to be and how what we did would impact upon Linda.

CHAPTER 10

"There, there...there, there..."

Just as there was no way for me to know, as 2021 was close to rolling into 2022, how spectacularly grueling the next few months would be for Linda, neither did I understand the terrible toll it would take on me. I think I may have been living in a pipe dream when I brought hospice aboard. There may have been more than a little idealizing of what I thought they could do for us. Why, I kidded myself, they'd lift most of the weight off my shoulders of hands-on caregiving! No more terrors. No more sleepless nights.

I'd read too much Dickens. There was Little Nell, suffering so nobly, so angelically, toward her inevitable death, or Dora Spenlow, the young and child-like first wife of David Copperfield, making of her death a virtual heavenly ascension while tacitly directing David toward the even more angelic Agnes Wickfield. Life isn't like that, as much as I might have wanted it to be. I'd been the one who insisted upon being there for Linda right to the end, with both of my hands all over her. After all, Linda had done exactly that for me when she was too young to understand what that effort would cost her—and it was still costing her. And my dogged insistence to stay the course with her fed directly into choosing for her the option of conducting hospice in our home, with me as a 24/7 amateur health provider. I absolutely know that I had only a foggy conception of what being there meant and would continue to mean two years beyond her death. But I was about to get a brutal dope-slap of a reality check. And I had it coming.

As luck would have it, I began keeping a rough running daily log of what was going on in Linda's bedroom, now a fully stocked hospital space. I hadn't read what I'd written since I made my last entry the night Linda died until the following day as I was agonizing over how I would represent those last few months. Beset sometimes with the curse of overstatement, a weak memory, and occasional misrepresentation, I knew I needed to rely on it to tell the truth of what happened. But I'm not so naïve as to think that what I'll translate here from what I scrawled illegibly back then can't, as Peruvian magical realist Mario Vargas Llosa explained in his *A Writer's Reality*, be more than a fictionalized version of reality. Nonetheless, it's all I've got and the best I can do. Donald J. Trump would love that—just a little high and outside of his labelling of journalism that trashes him as "fake news."

I've neglected to mention the bad stuff that began to happen just before the bed arrived on December 13. As my log had it, "Linda's sense of comfort begins, but not before a really difficult and terror-laden transfer to the bathroom and back." My sense of hospice as some kind of misty idyll seems reflected in what I wrote just a couple of hours later: "A second mattress equipped with air circulation comes, and we make the last bathroom transfer noisily. Linda eats comfortably in bed. She appears to be coping with the changes, although she did confide in me the question, 'What's happening?' She sleeps soundly." The next morning, "she has had cereal for breakfast and a slice of chicken pie for dinner."

But the following day proved to be much less idyllic:

A tough one for Linda. She had to put up, for a much longer time than should have been necessary, with the floundering of her husband and a young caregiver who hadn't performed the task of in-bed chuck-changing and the challenge of a full-on mega dump. We dropped the ball—and other things—for an unmercifully long time as we kept flipping Linda from side to side like a frying walleye. And you bet she howled and screamed. We eventually got it done, but at the expense of Linda's comfort. And it raised the as-yet unanswered question of how competent I'll be performing these challenging tasks alone this weekend. We've got the meds sorted out now. On a brighter note, I peaked in on Linda at 12:40am to a bright and lucid and cheerful "Hi...how are you doing?" And we had a little bright and lucid conversation, during which I expressed concern that she had completely uncovered herself and wasn't sleeping. She expressed frustration that she hadn't been able to sleep at all, but she wasn't unhappy or upset, and I found her in exactly the same sleepless cheerful state at 2:30am and 8am. It's going to be a challenging day for all of us this sleepy Thursday.

The lucidity and cheer had evaporated by Friday, the 17th, though:

> 'What's going on?' she fired at me. 'What's happening to me? Get me out of here!,' wherever 'here' was to her in that moment. Beginning to howl and writhe, she said, 'Why do I have to stay in this bed? When am I going to get better? Will it be years?' To which I responded 'no.' 'Then will it be many months?' she pressed. 'It will be months,' I said. She persisted: 'When will I get better?' 'It's a terminal illness, Linda,' I said softly. 'There's no getting better. That's what's so pernicious about this disease. So much of what I'll be paying attention to is if and when you are no longer interested in food—that's a bad sign. Remember when I and the hospice lady were talking about health directives and end-of-life issues? You were listening. I asked you if you were. Remember, there's always the chance that you'll be allowed out of hospice because you no longer fit their criteria. That's why I'm so

relieved that you're here with me until you aren't. I will always be there for you. And you probably won't remember much of this when you wake up tomorrow.'

What a guy. What an astounding bedside manner. I didn't believe much of any of this. Being there in that way, talking that way to her. I just didn't. It was surreal. And, yet, it had been a pretty good day otherwise. I'm feeling more competent now in changing her in bed. She used some drugs on the second change and that helped. Her attitude and internal strength had returned to very good.

December 18th brought more of the same, with Linda getting more curious about what was happening to her and where this was all going. Holding in her head what we'd talked about a day earlier was becoming increasingly difficult, although her steel-trap long-term memory hadn't lost a thing: "When am I going to get out of this bed? Why am I here? I hate this!" And, of course, she wasn't merely raving. Her intuition was right. I needed to push back against the idea that her mind was breaking up. I heard the glimmerings of the ability to think; that hasn't all gone away. It wasn't so good of a day. I had to change her three times in her bed alone. I came close to doing a competent job the third time, but it was still too much like practicing artificial respiration on a mannequin.

But the first two attempts took too long and unfolded like a bad Jerry Lewis comedy routine. And she hated Jerry Lewis. Linda was being very kind to me in my clumsiness, even including asking me if she had been screaming too loudly during the process. And, when I answered yes, she dialed it down. But she continued to be insistent about leaving the bed, and I tried to accommodate her by moving a chair beneath the bed rails so that, if she was successful in sitting up, she'd have a place to rest her feet. But the attempt to sit her up proved too painful for her, and I told her I was abandoning it for another time.

The next day we tried once more, to no avail. But she ate very well: a chocolate waffle for breakfast and Shrimp

Clemenceau for dinner, which she really liked. I felt badly about failing to get her up off her back. If it was even at all possible—and I'd need to be very careful with the catheter hose and bag—it would require two people.

At 9:20 pm at the end of a bleak and lonely Christmas Day, Linda started complaining, vigorously and loudly, about pressure on her chest, as if something was forcing her to cough. And cough she did, long and loud. Simultaneously, she doubled over while desperately claiming that she had to pee but couldn't. Her catheter bag was only a quarter full. The doubling-over and urgent coughing went on for about fifteen minutes. I gave her a vial of the morphine-based lorazepam, which seemed to kick in quickly. But, more to the point, what was the writhing and coughing all about? It wasn't nearly the first occurrence. Very anxiety producing, for her and for me.

On the evening of the 27th of December at about 9:10pm, I'd convinced Linda to accede to my turning off the TV on the dresser at the base of her bed and go to sleep. But, before that could happen, I'd need to check her chuck since she hadn't taken a dump since the day before. Suddenly, as I was gathering my materials and undoing the tape attached to Linda's inner thighs that held her catheter and hose securely in place to check her chuck, Linda became highly agitated and complained of pain. The pad revealed only a little soiling, but, as I began to roll a new chuck up and tuck it under her to remove the dirty one, the agitation exploded into panic. Fist-clenching on the right-side bed bar, prolonged screaming, followed by anxiety-driven coughing. And, just as suddenly, Linda exclaimed that she had to go. "Ok," I said, "take your time; everything is fine."

But, after five minutes and no apparent bowel relief, I tipped her up on her side to see if I could tell where the pain was coming from that was driving the screaming and coughing. And there it was—a bowel blockage, leaving a five-inch ball of crap stuck half-way out of her rectum. I was able to remove the blockage, which was then followed by an excremental explosion, thus relieving the pressure. But the pain continued for her through the completion of the chuck change, with no ostensible relief provided by the vial of lorazepam that I had administered at the onset of her agitation. And, even after cooling down for ten minutes, she said that she still felt pain, though much diminished. Very scary for her and for me.

She woke up the next morning looking incredibly exhausted from her ordeal. I made a promise to myself to give Linda a dose of lorazepam before retiring every night going forward. Nonetheless, she was spent and unresponsive all day in contrast to how alert and interactive she had been the day before leading up to the bowel event.

But it all came to a head at 5:30pm when Heidi set about freshening Linda up with a new chuck and pads—lots and lots of deafening screaming alternating with hysteria and uncontrolled coughing intermixed with a series of other wild noises. About a half-hour in, Heidi asked for my help to change Linda who, having become so excited, had blown by her catheter balloon twice and soiled two pads in a row with urine. Heidi succeeded on the third try, but the extreme agitation continued until we were finished. Heidi informed me that Linda's agitation had started before she was touched at all, and that had been true for me during the agitation on the previous night as well.

This behavior was clearly an escalation of anything we'd seen before, and it raised several questions: what was happening to her? Where was all of this going? Would it get worse and make it impossible for us to work with Linda? Would the bouts of terror and hysteria ultimately overcome her? How many doses of haldol and lorazepam could/should we give her, how often, and at what cost to her? And, suddenly recalling Yossarian's incompetence at the end of *Catch-22* and connecting it to the current exposure of mine, where are the Snowdens of Yesteryear?

December 29 was a terrible day from start to finish. And it would set the trend for all Linda's days going forward. It began with an exhausted woman lying mostly inert and unresponsive, and it went downhill fast from there. As she always did, Heidi began to freshen Linda up at the end of her shift at 5:30, and, after lots of screaming and delirium, I helped Heidi finish up, with some considerable difficulty, by 6:25. Fifty-five minutes to change a pad and chuck, with no bowel movement. That reflects the fierce level of Linda's agitation. That agitation continued unabated; the five milligrams of lorazepam hadn't made a discernible dent in it.

After Heidi left, and after realizing that Linda wouldn't be interested in eating, I succeeded in calming her to the point of sleep and left her alone until 9pm. I checked her pad then, felt her pain when the screaming resumed, and gave her another dose of lorazepam. That might have been enough to temporarily stop the screaming, but, when I closed the bedroom light, I knew the panic and terror would be flooding back later. I went to bed at 12:30 and didn't sleep, knowing what was surely coming.

It came at 3:10am. I'd asked Linda to call out to me should she need help, and call she did. From 3:10 to 4:45, Linda screamed, bellowed, coughed gutturally and spasmodically, writhed during what seemed like a delirious nightmare. Nothing to be done except to try to hold her flailing hand, mop her brow, quietly coach and reassure her, and sit in amazement at the incredible exertion she was expending.

By 3:15, I had phoned the night nurse, Carrie, at the hospice center. Under Carrie's direction, I started administering the three drugs available to me, and, very quickly, because it was Carrie's mission to help me stabilize Linda, she asked me to escalate those doses, but to no effect. Linda blew right through them, some of them four times the usual, causing us real concern. Carrie was mediating between me and our assigned hospice doctor as Linda kept on screaming and coughing scarily while hollering "no, no, no" and "ow-ow-ow."

After 4:45, Carrie stayed on the phone with me intermittently. She had told me that I probably had only two options: call 911, perhaps bringing more chaos to Linda by removing her to an ambulance and then on to the hospital, or keep escalating the meds in hopes that we'd be able to find the sweet spot to neutralize Linda's delirium. Kind of like trying to tranquilize a raging elephant.

By 6:35, the delirium began to subside, but only for thirty minutes, a brief respite until 7:10 after more drugs, and then another respite until 7:20, and then more drugs, including the delivery from the doctor of nitroglycerin, one tablet of which I gave to Linda, but to no effect. Unbelievable and deflating to those of us administering the stuff.

Carrie came back with a new plan: to come to our residence to check Linda's vitals and to observe what I'd been seeing. After 8:30 on the 30th, Carrie read me the tea leaves: since nothing was helping, she suggested checking Linda into the hospital's hospice section, where they could observe and monitor Linda and treat her in a professional and on-going way with the object of returning her home. I hated what I interpreted as intentionally using Linda as a yo-yo.

The other option, she said, was to keep her in her bed while introducing a couple of new drugs to move her to a point of stability. As it turned out, after several less explosive delirium fits, more and more drugs administered by Carrie at the recommendation of the doctor, Linda reached pacification by 10:15am. Carrie said that, in her thirty-five years of caring for people like Linda, she'd never seen anything like this. For the first time in seven hours, Linda was quiet and actually sleeping.

Then Carrie made a command decision: keep Linda home long enough to administer double doses of haldol every two hours to determine if she remained stable. She'd phone me at noon to see if there'd been a resumption of violent delirium, and, if so, for me to call the hospital to have Linda sent to the hospice unit. She remained quiet at noon, though, and again at 2pm after another double dose. My watch on Linda continued, with a hospice nurse scheduled to show up at 4pm to check on Linda. I waited with trepidation, wondering if I'd have another night with Linda like the previous one and, if not, how much morphine-based drugs would be needed to keep her pacified. What would Linda look like as a result?

By late afternoon, we'd determined a major reason for

Linda's delirium—a vaginal infection. Bad news under any circumstances, but awful for Linda. Another nurse was called in to mediate and consult with the doctor about how to proceed. Hospice had made crystal-clear their operating mission—to cease ancillary treatments to the admitted patient, put a stop on the patient's current medication list, and take no "extraordinary steps" or interventions to stop that patient's progress toward her inevitable end.

But there could be no choice. All people on Linda's case knew that a vaginal infection left untreated could kill her. The inflammation had blossomed and the pain had to have been unbearable. After some strained discussion, the doctor agreed that such an intervention was the only solution, particularly if hospice's mission to try to limit a patient's discomfort on the way to death had any true meaning. That meant bringing in the most experienced nurse to perform, with the help of Heidi, the procedure of removing Linda's catheter, taking extraordinary care in cleaning the area, and then installing a new one. How Linda howled amid a choir of comforting voices! I held her head and applied multiple doses of morphine-based drugs to try to ease her pain.

In the coming days, Heidi and I would need to be incredibly careful in cleaning and applying soothing cream around the area and to be on the alert for the pooling of urine around the catheter insertion site. This new catheter was equipped with a longer balloon, making the replacement even more painful. The color of Linda's urine had considerably darkened, meaning, as Heidi explained to me, that she hadn't been drinking enough water, and probably wouldn't in the days ahead. Obviously, killing the infection would require the use of antibiotics over the next several days, and we'd need to watch Linda carefully. The prospect of Linda not eating and drinking less spelled end-times.

So, there we were. A very crowded house of medical professionals, including Linda's case doctor, who prescribed three mgs of penicillin every hour for ten hours. She would revisit

Linda's dangerous situation late in the day of New Year's Eve. She moved the haldol doses from four vials to two every six hours and would monitor how that change worked on the 31st. We all continued to be concerned that Linda had not had a bowel movement for the previous four days, and that last one had been murder for her.

Then, on the 31st, a complication, this one not particularly medical. A new nurse entered Linda's room with a ton of experience and an attitude. We should all have been beyond expressing attitudes by this juncture. It should be evident that I had a big attitude of my own and got a little defensive when she questioned what Heidi and I had been doing in caring for Linda's infection. As she pushed back, I pulled rank on both her and Heidi and asserted, strongly but with no animus, that the focus had to be on Linda, not who was right. Remarkably, the nurse softened, admitting that she'd come on a little too strong, and things improved from there.

The major issue between us had been the UTI, and the new nurse, Annie, aggressively questioning why we were treating it. From her understanding, treating it posed more danger to Linda (she sited aspiration issues). I defended my decision to do it because the doctor had given the OK. My biggest concern was that the UTI had clearly been around for a while, the infection had worsened, and was most likely contributing to the delirium we'd been seeing. Annie had known none of that, apologized, and we proceeded to work together like fast friends.

So, we decided to wait on giving further doses of penicillin pending how Linda handled the new dosage adjustment of haldol to 1mg every six hours, but two mgs at bedtime and through the night as needed. Also, it was determined to give her one more dose of morphine to help her deal with the real reason Annie had arrived: to give Linda a suppository. That was a good thing because, though it caused Linda much discomfort, what with all the shifting and flipping of her to each side, we discovered a major leakage from Linda's vaginal area which required us to change the entire bed and bathe her.

Linda had settled down now, but we knew that the bowel movement that she would have to have would be difficult because of the impacted crap. We were dealing with the anticipations of that pain right then, and, at 1pm, I administered a mg of haldol. When the bowel movement came, it was hard, a partial blockage, and not nearly complete, but we were able to work it out and bring her to a stable point.

But we'd been warned (and this was the primary reason for the suppository) that blockages like this and undo effort on Linda's part to pass it could result in rectal prolapse. And it would soon. A new mechanical procedure for me to learn. At least we'd gotten her to drink some lemonade after the exertion!

By Saturday on New Year's Day, we were back on the three-day protocol to knock out the infection. She'd need to pursue it through the following Monday. Meanwhile, she was doing a mg of haldol every six hours and two mgs through the night. But she hadn't fully emptied the waste in her rectum yet, and she was experiencing great discomfort. Matt, the first male nurse we'd had, came by on Saturday morning to give her another suppository. Even more discomfort but no relief.

On Sunday, the time had arrived to act on Linda's bowel impaction, but Linda did it for us: an incredibly muddy mess, followed by a large rock-like piece. All of this occurred over the space of an hour. I was alone and called for two people to assist: Heidi, at home, and someone from the nursing line at the hospice center. When they arrived, they found Linda in distress. It took the three of us to get this job done, and during the process, Annie discovered that Linda's rectum had prolapsed. It happened twice; both times Annie was able to reinsert it. I gave Linda her first dilaudid, and it immediately gave her relief.

For the rest of the day Linda was calm, responsive, but very quiet. She managed to eat two saltines, a spoonful of my risotto, and drink a good amount of pink lemonade. She was doing as well as anyone could possibly expect and was demonstrating tremendous grit. We'd need to wait for Monday to get a read on where she might be in her journey to the end of the road.

On January 3rd, the end appeared near. Heidi and I were not reading much of an affect in Linda. She had developed a major pain on the right side of her neck area. Hospice had delivered some Aspercreme patches, but I couldn't quite apply them to the specific area in question. I'd shifted more blankets and a pillow to the painful side. Things were looking dark.

At the end of the third day of UTI medicine, the infection persisted. Both the back and front of Linda's body were extremely hot. She was perspiring profusely and showing us more confusion, no desire to ingest food (and it had been about nine days since she'd had much of anything). She was drinking only twenty-two ounces of fluid per day now. We'd started introducing MiraLAX to what we were able to get her to drink. She'd grown steadily quieter though she was still making eye contact. Her status had been reduced to a day-to-day proposition; she was descending to the bottom.

Linda had to endure still another terribly painful catheter replacement, performed by Christine with great difficulty. There are no words to express Linda's agony at having to suffer a re-insertion of that new catheter after it had fallen out, causing a small disaster among her bed clothes. The curve of Linda's terminal disease had not changed through it all.

My greatest concern now was Linda's meager ingestion of food. She'd been eating less and less daily, and that posed the most significant danger to the shortening of her life. It had been alarming to see Linda repeatedly refuse to eat all day, nearly every day. As of January 30, Linda had gone, over a four-day span, without food—completely for two of those days, with only a pierogi on one day and a small chunk of my birthday cake (she couldn't resist the whipped cream frosting), a tiny amount of ice cream, and a bite out of a donut on the other day. Literally unsustainable. We'd see going forward.

By mid-February, something indeed had changed, and not for the good. Over the previous week from February 4th and 5th the previous weekend and parts of the week before, Linda had enjoyed something of a winning streak. She'd been eating minimally a couple of times a day, she'd been alert, and acting like she knew where she was and what she was saying and doing.

But suddenly a switch flipped in her. Starting on Thursday and Friday, Linda began to show increased restlessness and anxiety that she even gave voice to. She started once again to speak weakly, often unintelligibly. She ate less, slept more (but lightly and fitfully), and expressed that she was beset with pain. I became concerned about that pain and where she said she was feeling it: her vagina.

The previous night, when I entered her room about 12:35am to give her a dose of haldol before I turned in, I found her huddling in pain. She called out loudly to me twice, "Help me!" Desperate. She described her pain level as a "9" and she located it internally in her vagina. I gave her a dilaudid for the first time in a couple of weeks with the haldol and then sat with her for the next seventy-five minutes, watching her every movement. She became quiet, but only barely asleep because she kept repeatedly opening her eyes. I changed her position to her left side with no positive result. At the end of seventy-five minutes, she indicated her pain level had dropped only slightly to an "8," but the pain had moved, she said, to her hips. I gave her a second dilaudid and made her as comfortable as I could, considered but decided against calling the hospice emergency number, and told her to call out "help" if she needed it.

She didn't, but, when I entered again that Sunday morning, February 13th, the first thing she said was that she was doing very badly. Lots of pain. It was back in the vagina. She complained of a headache as well. She'd eaten a substantial breakfast the previous morning, but she'd had no food since. She spoke very weakly and incoherently. I administered a third dilaudid on top of the haldol I'd given her at 7:30am, and I didn't feel good about the state she appeared to be in. She was clearly turning a corner into a darker place.

I must mention one thing more as I struggled against my own sleepless stupor: Linda reeked of urine. That smell was partially due to a catheter leak, and she was drenched between and under her legs due to the bending and floundering she'd been doing through the night. I carefully changed her top sheet, pad, and chuck. The bottom fitted sheet remained amazingly dry. I washed her down thoroughly with warm soapy water without a protest from her, and I changed her gauze dressings around her vagina that had become disgustingly wet. I greased her up with some soothing antiseptic cream before applying new dressings and some tape to hold them in place. As I worked, I marveled at how her skin remained as soft as it had been when she was eighteen, and I won't tell how I know if one should ask.

I noted that the catheter was draining adequately but that the bag wasn't any more than half-full, much less than the previous day's output. I'd need to alert the rest of the team about the need to monitor her for the possibility of another deadly UTI. But I was bowled over by what she whispered to me when I had finished cleaning her: "I feel nothing." Zero pain. Headache gone. Vaginal pain gone. She then went immediately to sleep. A small gift. I'd try when she awakened to get her to eat some breakfast.

Over the next three weeks, there was little to say about how she was faring daily. Most significantly, although Linda hadn't eaten much at all for three months, causing her body mass to shrink markedly, things changed on March 6th, a Monday. No food at all, and the no-food zone continued for the next twelve days, unabated, without exception. So, on Saturday, March 18, Linda continued her no-food intake regime. No nutrients. Very concerning for those like me standing anxiously by to help her. Before March 6th, I could count upon her asking for chocolate milk, delivered to her in a glass through a straw. But her interest in chocolate milk had all but stopped, with one small exception of a syringe-full to help her wash down her medications. When I continued to offer it, she faintly whispered no or barely shook her head.

Hospice folks had told me that the cessation of eating, under her medical circumstances, was "normal," but it's painfully hard to accept. Hers was becoming a slow forced march to the only possible exit. Of course, the door remained open for her to request anything she could swallow and ingest and then safely pass down her throat. And that, said hospice, was a major concern, almost eliminating dairy products from the list of possibilities (and her inability to swallow would ultimately be the thing that killed her). Apple sauce, jello, some puddings, perhaps a well-scrambled egg.

But none of those options mattered anyway—she wasn't interested. And, more crucially, she was beginning to resist water intake, particularly ever since she had been made to take it through a ten ml syringe. This became the most dreadful aspect of Linda's fast as she rapidly weakened, shed weight and mass, and gradually lost the ability to move her limbs or to allow others to move and shift her in bed without causing her great pain.

And that left Heidi and me little to do but sit and watch her decline. There would be no reward for her to last longer, to persevere. And every morning she awoke again was merely another Pyrrhic victory, postponing the inevitable. I'm sadly reminded of the song, "Should I stay or should I go?" Well, there was no either/or about it for Linda. She had weakly cast her oral vote to us— "help me get up...help me out of here;" a defiant and still aware "I'm not dead yet...I want to leave!"

And I was increasingly with her on that. Of course, I ached for her to stay with me, but not like this. And, besides, Linda was no longer fully Linda anymore. Last week, after moving my mattress to the floor to sleep beside her bed (and I use the term "sleep" to refer to lying down with my eyes pinned open and my mind racing), I could look over and see her eyes wide-open, all through the night.

But, after the 18th, sleep was all she was doing. A preview of coming attractions. She had become inert, still a beautiful woman transformed into a pretty rag doll, her voice nearly inaudible, her faintly spoken words so difficult to understand because her tongue barely functioned, her eyes narrowing to tiny slits, her breathing soft but quickening, the apnea she experienced becoming far more frequent and sometimes disturbingly long.

Clearly, Linda's end was standing in the doorway. I vowed, amid the Christmas lights that provided the only light in her room to watch her, to never remove them. The tree in the living room that she'd never seen, decorated with so many of the precious ornaments and birds that she'd so lovingly purchased, would stay up for another year until I reluctantly took it down.

But the end, for her and for me, would be frustratingly indefinite. I'd been told what to look for, and that's what I'll be writing about very soon. I've come to know Alzheimer's as the cruelest of afflictions. It refused to let go of her. Heidi and I had been seeing the skin-color changes, the waxiness, the deepening and purpling of her eye sockets, the alternating heat and cold that her body was enduring, the sudden tremors in her body and limbs that suddenly overtook her like electric shocks. There were no more bowel movements, no expulsion of gas as we shifted her to her side. It was unimaginable that she could persist, but she did. I didn't want her to go, and I couldn't imagine going on without her. But I rooted for her to do so. Just when one thinks that what one had been watching was too much, there was more. And there we were, on Dylan's "Watch Tower."

Assuredly, I thought, by the evening of March 19th, this must be the penultimate beginning of the end. I'd delivered three to four doses of heavy meds every four hours to Linda, with no water taken with them. *None.* She couldn't live without water. Oh, sure—she was beginning her fourteenth day of fasting, and, granted, I've heard of fasts that have lasted three weeks before intervention, but there would be no intervening here, by hospice's definition and my agreement.

Besides, Linda had entered this fast already fasting! That is, she had had no more than one small meal on any of the previous seven to eight days, and she had already been in a perilously weakened state. She was respiring at twenty-three to twenty-eight half-breaths per minute, very quickly. She was, to the human voice or touch, unreachable. Incommunicado. Beyond the pale, as my Irish forbears were wont to say. Wherever she was, she was not with me, and I didn't believe she was coming back. I was afraid to move her, to shift her weight to her other side by pulling on the chuck and then forcing a small pillow under her buttock. Any movement was painful to her now. I heard a faint moaning as I tried to re-position the pillow under her head. As I stood guard on the Watch Tower, I could barely make out the shape and sounds of the rider drawing closer.

It was Sunday, March 20th, and here we were. It had been a difficult night for Linda. Listening to her from my bed on the floor all night long, I'd heard what sounded for all the world like a person running a full marathon, with all of the attendant labored breathing. Through the night, the pace had been accelerating. Since 7am and now at 11am, although no one but my dad could ever have called me a quitter, I dearly wished that Linda would drop out of the race. She could not win. There was only one finish line for her to cross, and she ought to get to choose it. The respiration rate had climbed, minimally now, to thirty-five, a punishing pace of half-breaths. The speed of her breathing moved me to change her position a bit, getting her flat on her back with her head tilted more upright with a little pillow to support it. Because she was leaking a bit, I washed her soaked top sheet and the still chocolate milk-stained dog blanket that had served her so well. I carefully gave her fresh linens along with freshening her thigh and vaginal area.

She was ready for the stretch run now. I discerned what sounded like a distant occasional rattle in her throat between those rapid respirations. I put in a call to the day nurse to ask if doses of dilaudid every hour might serve to slow her breathing, and she gave me the go-ahead. But her breathing was still extremely quick, and she was beginning to gasp. Strange sounds were beginning to rise from her throat to interrupt her breathing as if she was trying to force air through a wet rag. This couldn't go on for long. It was nearing the spring clean for the May Queen. As Linda's half-breaths rose to an impossible rate of fifty-eight per minute, I called Karen and asked if she wanted to be with her mom in her final moments.

But she arrived too late to see what I saw—the sudden opening of Linda's eyes. She looked directly at me and seemed to smile slightly, her final gift to me. Her breathing slowed over a few minutes as I tried to reach her and comfort her. And then, at 6:30pm after a day-long expense of all her resources, she slightly rolled her head toward me, closed her eyes, and left.

"Love alters not with his brief hours and weeks but bears it out even to the edge of doom."[4]

---

[4] Shakespeare's *Sonnet 116* (1609).

CHAPTER 11

An Interview With Karen

So, here, at last, we were, some two years after Linda's death, having finally reached the point of my interview with my intrepid daughter Karen. Months ago, when I had broached the prospect of writing about her mom's illness and the horrible way that it ended, I warned her that I would emphatically need her not merely to verify where she could what I had experienced over the years of mom's mental decline but also to fill in the blanks that only she could fill in her close and sometimes problematic interactions with her over the years when I wasn't present and to challenge some of my assumptions with experience that would frankly contradict it.

It's probably useful here to remember what I'd hoped to discover in the process of writing this book. Were there predispositions genetic in a person toward dementia and/or Alzheimer's, and could I reasonably track some of that in Linda through what I'd be able to rediscover about her mom? Might I be able to point to any evidence in the kinds of exposures, incidents, aspects of upbringing, and established dietary habits that might make dementia or Alzheimer's more likely in a person like Linda? Can enduring a "not good enough mother" make one more vulnerable to early-onset dementia and Alzheimer's—that is to say, a mother incapable of providing an unrelenting, secure, and caring "holding environment" through the early crucial years of ego-identity formation[5]? And, most importantly, could a series of traumas experienced by a child and then as a mature adult cause a person to be more likely to develop dementia or Alzheimer's?

I knew before the interview even began that it wouldn't be easy or pleasant. There was even a good chance that it would never occur. Karen had already begged off once from a scheduled date with reasonable claims of interference with her busy schedule of tennis practices, matches, and doctor appointments. And, in the messages that the two of us exchanged, it became clear that this would be difficult for Karen. It didn't seem like two years since we had lost Linda, and her final two weeks had been excruciating to watch and participate in, as Karen had.

But there was more to it that made a discussion about her relationship with her mom difficult. There had been issues between them over the years that had made their relationship tense and often combative. Karen and her mom, it seemed, had some prolonged and unresolved issues. I loved them both unreservedly, but, once more, my narcissism blinded me. If something going on in the family didn't have to do directly or indirectly with me, my professional identity, or my work, I was more likely to see right past it or not to hear it.

As it turned out, I didn't know half of what was going on with them. Par for the course. Just like me: tuning things out that didn't have to do with me. But I'd been forewarned: Karen had told me before we met for the interview that she'd been concerned about saying anything about her mom that would upset me or make me feel badly about the woman I'd lived with for fifty-seven years. It wouldn't take long for me to realize that

---

[5] See D.W. Winnicott's discussion of "the good enough mother" in *Playing and Reality* (Abingdon-on-Thames: Routledge Classics, 2005), 144-48. All subsequent references to Winnicott's book will be made parenthetically a *DWW#*.

what she might be inferring was code for my obliviousness.

I was anxious as I awaited her arrival at my second floor flat on an uncommonly warm late afternoon in February. I'd even vacuumed, made coffee, and bought some brie. I felt a certain hesitancy and resistance from Karen earlier in the week, and I'd need to tread lightly and find an icebreaker to ease her into it. I'd spent a good amount of time developing, polishing, and sequencing the thirty questions I'd formulated for her—so similar to the way I used to prepare for my own job interviews so many years before! And maybe it was I who was the subject of this interview. I had intended the questions to focus on the two testing and evaluating sessions by Dr. Fuhrman and Linda that Karen and I had attended years earlier. I'd even sent the questions to Karen via e-mail enclosure the previous day to try to take the edge off any anxiety she might be feeling.

I'd never told her so—it's ironic that Karen knew it already and would tell me so explicitly during the interview—but I'd made Karen my confidante through so much of Linda's illness. She had become a far less myopic second pair of eyes as well as ears that didn't suffer from hearing loss. Throughout our journey into Linda's illness, even though she hadn't been constantly present, she had been positioned to confirm or deny important parts of Linda's story as told from my perspective.

But, more than that, she knew much more about Linda's illness through her informal and focused research than I ever would. She might well serve as the rational voice that could talk me down from what I believed had precipitated Linda's fall into dementia and ultimately Alzheimer's. I needed to know if mom shared with her (and, if not with her, then no one!) anything about the "big three" traumas occurring consecutively, in fairly rapid fire that sent her into a largely silent downward spiral, almost as if she'd been the victim of three separate, severe, and repeated major concussions without any opportunity to recover from one head injury before the violent application of the next one. We're talking cumulative trauma here; more on that later.

No sooner had Karen entered my flat and sat down than

my long list of prepared questions got thrown up in the air and discarded. After apologizing for anything she might say that could upset me, she plunged ahead into what would be a forthright and unsparing analysis of her understanding of her mom and their relationship.

Karen was ready and eager to talk and needed little prompting. There was a kind of chaos to our conversation, but consistent themes ran through it. Karen immediately characterized her overall experience with mom as "emotionally stunted." Karen recollected Linda, from her interactions with her in her middle and high school years, as incapable of managing and processing her emotions. There were many arguments, ones that rarely resolved into a satisfying conclusion. As Karen put it, "she was 'unavailable' to me." Rather than being able to work through a disagreement rationally, Linda would explode, abruptly remove herself from any given argument, inappropriately make it all about herself, and then run to her bedroom and slam the door. There were too many situations when Karen was left on the other side of that door listening to her mother crying inconsolably.

After struggling through her recollection of incidents like these, Karen concluded that her mom shut down because she had been unable to confront what she felt. I had been privy to a number of these sharp clashes between mother and daughter, but I'd found them unremarkable and brushed them aside as the push and pull that occurs normally between parent and adolescent. But Karen wasn't having any of that. She gleaned something competitive in their friction. Whether it was Karen or Chris that was her opponent, the result was nearly always a meltdown, leaving either Karen or Chris responsible for it.

And mom never apologized for her part in the arguments. Instead, Karen said, the stress in the parent-child relationship continued to grow. Karen remembered—and I can attest to it—how unrebellious she had been as a teenager. No drinking, smoking, drugging, getting into trouble, running away from home (Chris had shown just a little of this, even absconding with our car for a few hours before calling us from Duluth to ask if it would be okay if he came home). This was a smart, consistently dutiful young woman with good judgement, lots of friends, and strong motivation to succeed. No maladjustments nor lack of motivation here. In fact (and she said as much to me), with all the difficulties that her mom was having controlling her emotions, Karen could be said to have nearly brought up herself.

I was shocked when Karen recalled being put in the position at seven of being a latch-key kid, and she had been frightened by that. All of that transpired in the winter and spring of 1980 after I'd taken a one-year replacement position at the College of St. Benedict in St. Joseph, Minnesota. This was a low point for our little family. We'd rented a large home in the little hamlet of Avon about twelve miles from campus and directly fronting the loud north-bound portion of four-lane I-94 heading toward North Dakota. The town had scarcely five hundred souls living in it. The unattractive and unmythical Lake Woebegone lay directly across the street.

We had taken up residence there about nine years before the eleven-year-old Jacob Wetterling would be abducted at gun point by a sexual predator just before dark close to the little abbey and campus of St. Ben's. Of course, I was teaching at the college for criminally small money. When Linda was offered a temporary full-time teaching position in the adjoining town of New Albany, from January to June, we irresponsibly entrusted little Karen with the care of our barely one and a half year-old Chrstopher until I or Linda could escape from our jobs and return home in early afternoon. We had little money for childcare beyond what we paid a woman down the street to look after Chris until Karen could rescue him in early afternoon after she'd arrived home on the bus. We paid Karen a quarter an hour to watch Chris and care for his needs. Even while frightened by the responsibility, Karen felt "a sense of pride that she'd been entrusted" to look after her baby brother. And regardless of what one could say about her parents' part in all of this, she carried it all off brilliantly.

For whatever reason, Karen had sensed shame and guilt at the core of Linda's failure to work through her relationship with her. Because of that failure, in Karen's words, "mom saw herself as 'a bad person.'" And that shame and guilt exposed itself with every long-distance phone call that her mother Dorothy made to her. Karen was there to answer those calls on many occasions; invariably, the first words "Gramma" spoke to her daughter were, "how much do you weigh" and "what size are you wearing now?" Always judgements, followed by Dorothy's passive-aggressive disparagements and points of comparison with her own weight. The inevitable result of these calls and the bad feelings they always produced were the consequent pushing of Karen's buttons by Linda. According to Karen, "she felt ashamed of who she was in her mother's eyes."

Karen has had a long time to think about her relationship with her mom, particularly in relation to her own parenting. Some ten years ago, a large house that she and her husband Hunter had purchased caught fire in the early morning hours. As Hunter was leaving for work, he'd looked back and seen smoke emanating from the garage soffits and raced back to alert Karen and their two children. The fire department had been busy answering another alarm and were late in arriving at what was now a full-blown blaze over the garage and the upstairs portion of the house, but the water damage resulting from extinguishing the fire turned the house into a total loss.

From the conclusion of that traumatic event and their thoughts of how much more they could have lost, each of the four family members entered psychological therapy, and they have continued that therapy to this day. For the kids as well as the parents, regularized therapy and the ability to talk to a professional in a secure and private space has been particularly beneficial in helping each of them through the anxieties brought to the surface by the fire and their necessary adjustments to difficult parental and family challenges as their two kids have confronted major identity issues through and beyond their teenage years,

Karen has grown tremendously through her many years of therapy. That's also true about the understanding she's reached about her relationship with her mother and the anxieties and compulsions that bedeviled her. One thing both Karen and I remember about Linda was her practical problem-solving ability. So much more than I, Linda could fix anything mechanical or electrical. Her problem-solving expertise extended from building multi-shaped containers, both metal and wood, to contain her wide variety of beads, fasteners, and cutting and shaping tools to developing a perfect understanding of how to pack and tie down materials to fit into any container up to a huge moving van. She understood space and how to fill it, and it became a near compulsion for her.

Karen particularly remembered her birthday celebrations, how her mom would make all the cards and decorations. And there was always a remarkably creative cake. One of her most vivid recollections was a birthday in Evansville, Indiana, in 1979 when Karen was six. Linda had made the theme of the party "Holly Hobby" at the time when that doll was so popular. Of course, Linda had custom-made a Holly Hobby bonnet for each of Karen's friends as well as a cake shaped and colored and frosted into a perfect representation of Holly Hobby, In some ways, it seemed all about being competent to Karen; Linda had had to learn to be from a very early age due to her mother's practiced indolence and the pressure to do the practical things that her mother wouldn't. I was surprised to hear Karen say, "I should always be dutiful and not make my mom cry," which caused me to flash back to what Linda had told me about needing always to perform the duties that Dorothy had prescribed to avoid being beaten by her mother's wooden hairbrush.

Karen's therapy had provided her with the distance to understand why she had struggled so with her mom. Linda had taken a rooting interest early in Karen's senior year in high school as Karen labored through the college application process. Through her talent, Karen was accepted at all five of the best schools she'd applied to. As she and I visited four of the schools in New England before she settled on her final choice, Linda clearly gained some extra pride in conveying Karen's success to

Dorothy, rubbing her nose in it perhaps because Dorothy had never gone to college and, from my personal knowledge, had no expectation or desire that Linda ever would.

Linda was an overachiever—not just in the sense of having to overcome others' low expectations of what she could do or having to work harder to succeed. But it was easy to see how external stimulation from an attachment outside her nuclear family (usually me) could and did spur her to reach beyond what other significant people in her life seemed convinced she was capable of. And, once she'd acted on that encouragement, she would not quit until she'd succeeded, even if it meant that she'd have to suffer pain and even embarrassment in the process. I point to Linda's refusal to quit school during her first three semesters due to borderline grades while she was caring for me during my long recovery from injuries from a car accident as well as her refusal to turn down job-ending lap years at Viterbo and Augsburg despite the real humiliation she must have experienced. Stunning.

That's why I think, though Karen might disagree, that Linda pushed her daughter hard to be able to compete for admission into elite schools. Linda was no helicopter parent—she never interfered with or managed Karen's accomplishments and choices. But there couldn't have been anyone prouder of Karen's performance in the classroom, at dance recitals, and in her stage performances.

That probably accounts for the delight that Linda exuded when, after losing some seventy-five pounds, looking like a twenty-five-year-old, and feeling as good about herself as she had in years, she went alone to visit Karen for several days at Bryn Mawr College outside Philadelphia. Karen recalled her mom showing up energetic and enthusiastic about Karen's living situation and her roommates. But Karen viewed that visit differently. Yes, mom had a great time, Karen confirmed, but largely because, as Karen perceived it, mom spent the bulk of her time trying to be helpful to everyone. As Karen put it, "mom's value came from what she did for others…Mom was useful, and that made her feel good."

As I think back over my life with Linda, I find myself concurring with Karen's observation. Linda lived a life of dedicated service to me, the kids, the various churches we belonged to, the schools that the kids attended. Often, as I recall, her willingness, almost compulsion, to serve was taken advantage of. She knew it; nonetheless, she did it anyway.

It is beyond odd to me that Karen vividly remembered her mom's efforts to do laundry, clean, and help Karen's roommates in as many ways as she could while having no other recollection of her being there. No real intimate, loving interactions. Although I put the question to her repeatedly, Karen was unable to provide any "feel-good" memories of her mom. All of her "kid memories had been complicated, she said, maybe even compromised, by mom's situational responses: "If she praised me, it felt almost like a comparison that was a judgement of herself…mom would make it about her. She couldn't help herself." Regarding the Bryn Mawr visit, it became clear to Karen that mom "wanted some of the limelight," but her efforts to gain positive attention from Karen's friends subtracted from Karen: "It wasn't a feel-good situation." Karen's reaction to that visit needs to be compared to how Linda described it to me with nothing but satisfaction and superlatives.

Linda could not see herself as Karen saw her. Or, perhaps, she couldn't allow herself to do so. When Karen was very young, she remembers her mom "making stuff for me that wasn't always what I wanted." It was a crushing blow to Karen—and to me when she told me—about her direct experience of having mom as a "sub" in her school, and it would happen frequently. When Karen entered junior high, she caught an ear-full from other students about "how mom was hated by nine and ten year-olds" because of her severe demeanor. That wasn't always the way Linda's classroom was evaluated when she taught many years earlier at the elementary school level, and, after all, being a sub and maintaining control of an unruly class not her own altered the equation.. But Linda had grown up through the "old school" approach to class discipline, and it had fallen out of favor. Karen remembers ducking her head in embarrassment to avoid her fellow students making the connection between her and their temporary teacher. There was an inflexibility to Linda by this time, and not only in the classroom, that she could not see, never mind soften,

That brittle inflexibility expressed itself against another person that Karen had held in high regard—my Aunt Ellen. I'd had a long, rocky relationship with Ellen over the years. For reasons that remain unclear to me, Ellen believed me to have become a grade-A juvenile delinquent, disappointing parents by traveling with bad people, stealing cars, getting into fights, and engaging in other anti-social behaviors. To be honest, I had gotten into some minor trouble. I'd participated in taking a car not my own for a joy ride through Boston, and some of my friends were sketchy. Since my mother had been stricken with cancer, I'd fallen into a rebellious phase. However, from what I could determine, most of the things Ellen blamed me for in nasty phone calls to my parents' home were a combination of hearsay and projection from her son onto me as a way of masking his own bad behavior.

But over the years, after my parents had died, we warmly reconciled and, when my kids were old enough, Linda and I introduced them to Ellen. Chris was just an infant then, but Ellen and Karen immediately and lovingly bonded. Because we lived over a thousand miles away from Ellen's big house perched on the side of a steep hill in Quincy, Massachusetts, our visits with the loud and demonstrative Ellen didn't occur often, but, when they did, Ellen was ready with a decorated house, lots of games and toys she'd purchased for the occasion, and a baby grand that Karen got to play—brim full of love and genuine enthusiasm. And her two grown boys Allan and David loved her too. It didn't matter when our visits occurred—Ellen would entertain the kids at the soda fountain in the health and beauty aids store she managed and later on her front porch as she launched bottle rockets, sparklers, and cherry bombs over the roofs of adjoining houses. A real piece of work she was, and Karen loved her despite Ellen and my Uncle Billy being raging alcoholics.

For whatever reason, Linda remembered all of the bad things about Ellen—her bad-mouthing me years earlier; the frequent transparent visits to the kitchen to down straight shots of whiskey before returning to try to preserve her convincing act of sobriety; Ellen's larger-than-life tough-talking and belly-laughing; and the unforgettable hour of bridge we tried to play with Ellen and a sodden, profane Uncle Billy before the game collapsed into chaos and name-calling. This was a brief and violent recital of what their forced marriage, hateful relationship, and Billy's descent into full-time inebriation driven by his disappointment of being no more than a car salesman at his father-in-law's Buick dealership that he'd fully expected to be groomed to take over. Ellen never stopped loving him despite the indignities and insults he made her suffer through and willingly followed Billy down the alcoholic drain.

But, to give her credit, she somehow remained mostly fully functioning, kept her truant older alcoholic son within her reach long enough to see him succeed as a programmer and apartment building owner, and always held a job to pay the bills and even train her youngest son to learn the health and beauty aids retail business well enough to become a valued buyer for a major company.

By the time that she'd turned eighteen, Karen knew all of this, and, when Linda began to obliquely disparage Ellen, Karen saw that as meanness. She never forgot that expression of meanness nor the many kindnesses that Ellen had paid to both her and Chris. Karen understood that my family had largely become alienated from our relatives. She remembered Ellen as the only bright light in a fractured extended family that welcomed her in and showed her real love. When Ellen died suddenly around 1991 at age sixty-two, Linda couldn't rationalize the sadness Karen told me she felt at her passing,

I suspect that part of Karen's sadness derived from what she felt her mom had been too often unable to provide her with—openness, availability, and affection. Karen remembered Linda's defensiveness that she characterized as "like a trapped animal" which she speculated may have come from "a lot of self-loathing." It was no secret to Karen that "she felt ashamed of who she was in her mother's eyes." Linda expressed that shame in many ways; it often drove her, to eat what she knew she shouldn't, to reach into her purse for treats while doing errands with the kids and making them promise not to tell on her.

It's important to stop here for a moment and declare without reservation that Karen truly loved her mom, was shaken nearly as much as I was at her precipitous mental and physical decline, her awful night terrors, her three months of visibly wasting in bed while clinging to a sense of humor and some moments of mental sharpness, and a horrible death that looked and sounded like a slow drowning or oxygen starvation. Karen was there immediately after Linda's death, helping me to clean her body and remove the bed clothes. Always the dutiful, caring daughter. And she deeply mourned as I did.

But Karen's years of therapy, some of which had been spent on rediscovering who her mom had and had not been for her had helped her to see some things about her mom that had left a mark on her. She'd come to see her mom as a bridge-burner: "that's mom--when there's an argument or an impasse, mom burned it to the ground. When things didn't go well, she'd give you a 'fuck you' and run away."

Karen recalled vividly that, when the assisted living residence where Linda had placed Dorothy called to tell us that she had died, "mom was flippant and detached from any emotion." She was erecting a defense to protect herself, to be sane, but her reaction told us so much more about a failed, dismal, and ruinous mother-daughter relationship. She never openly grieved for her loss. Linda, Karen mused, was "starved for her mother's approval and never got it." When Linda had been dealt heavy blows—both physical and psychological—by a mother who'd been unable to express her love to her, "she didn't have the capacity to take care of herself. She hadn't learned the skills," and, consequently, couldn't pass them on to Karen.

And then Karen surprised me with some illuminating information about mom's entrance into a woman's change of life. I guess I vaguely knew that Linda experienced some extreme reactions when menopause began for her. There were whiplash mood changes and the most severe hot flashes. I remembered vaguely that Linda had become more difficult to get along with without having any clear idea of when she began to experience these changes. That's why I was shocked to learn from Karen that Linda had begun menopause so early—between thirty-nine and forty. Along with everything else she was struggling with— fruitless attempts to get a public-school teaching job; her constant battle with weight; the insoluble love/hate war with her mother fought occasionally during Dorothy's visits to our home in Mankato with Dorothy playing the passive-aggressive victim while Linda exploded (I can still hear Linda's high-pitched rageful rants at Dorothy while mowing the front lawn).

Suddenly, Linda's body was betraying her. Not long after that, perhaps in 1988 in her forty-second year when she had launched into her Ph.D. program in Curriculum and Instruction at the University of Minnesota and was living part-time in an off-campus apartment owned by two teaching colleagues from Mankato State, Linda began to experience severe abdominal pain. Upon further examination, her physician discovered horrible fibroids in her uterus, and almost immediately she was prepped for a full hysterectomy. Ironically, Karen related that, at some later point, Linda discovered from Dorothy that she, too, had suffered from fibroids but had neglected to inform her. For the next thirty years, Linda would continue to experience the unrelenting agony of hot flashes.

Shortly after her recovery from her hysterectomy in mid-1988, after my many vigorous attempts to convince her to find a therapist to talk through her several difficulties, Linda finally agreed. Both Karen and I concurred that her engagement with a female therapist in Mankato was a brief one, lasting no longer than six to nine months. She didn't share much with me about those sessions—only that she had gained some measure of relief from them. Interestingly, Karen told me something else I didn't know but could easily infer, that mom was diagnosed with depression by her therapist. "Mom told me," Karen said," but Chris never knew." Soon, though, Linda's therapist left town to take another position, and, though Karen and I separately urged her to continue therapy and find another psychologist she could confide in, Linda adamantly refused. Karen's speculation about why her mom would shut down and go silent over even the suggestion of returning to therapy—that "she stopped emotionally maturing at a point where her needs were never met"—might be pertinent.

From 1988 onward, Linda's life in and outside our home was becoming increasingly congested with higher-level course work to be completed, a semester-long study of the use of collaborative learning with the use of computer technology, and, after the granting of her degree, assembling a dossier and mounting a job search. That's the approximate time when, as Karen stipulated, anxiety began to become as much an issue for Linda as her depression. Was she good enough at what she was pursuing to do the work, complete and write up her research study to the point of approval, and compete successfully for a job after completing her program at the age of forty-six, never mind being able to overcome feelings of guilt she felt for the time she'd be spending away from a son who was now fourteen?

A heavy load to bear that would soon swing from accomplishment to rejection. Karen saw mom wanting to head off rejection and hurt in her personal relationships "by shutting the door on them," rather than the other way around. But soon she'd find herself unprepared for the shock of rejection that came from what others had concluded about her that she could not see.

After the trifecta of humiliations that Linda had endured through the 1990s, Karen had tried to get Linda to talk about them and about how badly they'd hurt her, but, true to form, "she pushed back hard." And from that point, with few exceptions, until nearly twenty years later, Karen became accustomed to Linda's growing passivity, disinterestedness in life around her, an enveloping inertia. Karen had been aware of Linda's decreasing mobility, of her discarding her cane for a wheelchair, and her frequent lapses into repetition in her speech.

She was cognizant of Linda's mental decline, but she wasn't prepared for what would unfold in August of 2017. I'd gone to the cabin about two hundred and forty miles away on the 10th to do some upkeep and gain a bit of distance from Linda's worsening situation that had led me finally to enlist some paid care-giving help. I'd no sooner arrived than I received an urgent call from Karen to return immediately. Linda had "fallen," or, as we'd soon be accustomed to describing it, slid from her upholstered chair to the area rug beneath it. Linda had not been hurt; having grown too heavy and weak from inactivity to climb back in the chair, Linda instructed her caregiver to call Karen, who quickly called the Fire Department, who then rushed over from the station located a mere street away and re-positioned her in her chair after checking her over for injuries.

But, although this wasn't the first call to the Fire Department, it was the first for Karen, and she was alarmed. As I rushed home, Karen tended to mom, now realizing from Linda's state of confusion and incoherence just how far Linda had declined. Karen called me again to tell me that she was driving mom to the hospital in St. Louis Park and for me to meet her there. When I arrived, Linda had already been assigned a room and had begun a series of tests that would extend over several days of observation. Our meeting with the neurologist Dr. Fuhrman was not many weeks away now, but Karen had begun to see, from her distanced perspective, a cluster of behaviors in her mom that I'd taken for granted from being too close and seeing her every day. Karen reminded me of how she'd gotten into my face and scorched me for refusing to "believe that mom couldn't be alone anymore" without me present.

The hospital stay didn't do much more than indicate elevated blood pressure and a deficit of oxygen along with confirmation of Linda's mental slippage, but, from that point onward, I made sure that there was always caregiver coverage for Linda and, if I had to be away from her overnight, there would always be someone staying with her with a monitor charting her breathing and alerting the caregiver if she should awaken, attempt to leave the bed by herself, or fall.

Karen could do what her mom had lost the will or ability to do—talk openly and assertively about Linda's mental decline. I think Linda was just a little afraid of that assertiveness, at the same time feeling great pride in the person that Karen had become. She could see what I couldn't or wouldn't and never hesitated to tell me so.

CHAPTER 12

A Broken Heart—The Most Likely Conclusion? [6]

Not long after Linda's series of traumas, she lost much of her willingness to "play," and, over time, she lost it all. Again, as Winnicott stipulates, play must be "spontaneous" (68). "Only in being creative" can "the individual discover the self" (*DWW* 73). In discarding those activities that once joyfully expressed Linda's creativity, she would lose herself.

What Winnicott says about how trauma or loss, untreated, can cause the creative self to weaken seems particularly pertinent to Linda's situation. Unable to find relief from the constant pain she suffered from her back operations and unsuccessful knee replacement surgeries, she gradually withdrew from her book

---

[6] Articles abound about the "broken heart" phenomenon. See "Broken Syndrome (takotsubo cardiomyopathy)" in https://www.health.harvard/edu-heart/jun13,2023 and "Broken heart syndrome – Symptoms and causes" from the Mayo Clinic in https;//www.mayoclinic.org/diseases-conditions/nov11,2023

club and craft work that had provided enrichment to her life. Although it's impossible to say to what degree the beginnings of dementia might have been responsible for her withdrawal from living to a state of apathy, occasionally there were glimmers of a buried secret life. As Winnicott says,

> One has to allow for the possibility that there cannot be a complete destruction of a human individual's capacity for creative living and that, even in the most extreme case of compliance and the establishment of a false personality, hidden away somewhere there exists a secret life that is satisfactory because of its being creative or original to that human being. Its unsatisfactoriness must be measured in terms of its being hidden, its lack of enrichment through living experience. (*DWW* 92).

Even as her control of her bodily functions progressively diminished and her world shrank, Linda continued, in her silent way, to work through an endless number of coloring books, emerge from watching me and her favorite caregiver doing jigsaw puzzles to insert the occasional puzzle piece, and ask me to read to her (Austen's *Pride and Prejudice* and, somewhat ironically, *The Perfect Storm* were particular favorites). Her inner self was hidden but not out of reach.

Winnicott's student, friend, and patient M. Masud Khan has written extensively about the hidden self, tracking and then interpreting the dream-texts of several of his patients in *The Privacy of the Self* [7]. Though I don't mean to establish a direct connection between Khan's work on dreams and the effects of Linda's several psychic traumas spanning from the sudden violent death of her father, her having been uprooted from all that had been happy and familiar, a confused relationship with a depressed and narcissistic mother, to her diminished mental state toward the end of her life, one of Khan's dream spaces seems to

---

[7] M. Masud R. Khan, *The Privacy of the Self: Papers on Psychoanalytic Theory and Technique* (New York: International Universities, Inc., 1974). Subsequent references to this book by Khan will be made parenthetically by: PRIVACY #.

resonate with the quiet, withdrawn person she was near the end.

What follows is a complete text of one of Khan's female patients:

> "...about my mother carrying my father's coffin downstairs. I was standing to one side at the bottom of the stairs and was upset to see that his head had to be in a separate coffin and that both coffins were so thin. I wondered how they'd managed to get his body in and thought his feet must have been hurt in getting them to lie flat. My mother opened the coffin with his head in—it looked like a cold joint of meat—skull-shaped—and my mother got a knife and made an incision where the nose would have been and then scrubbed on a place on his cheek till some of the flesh came up. Then she put two apples in one eye socket. While this ritual was going on, I felt very miserable and watched my tears sinking into the carpet..." (*PRIVACY* 206-07)

In his interpretation of the dream, Khan hones in on the patterns of alienation it exhibits: the daughter's almost clinical detachment from the unfolding ritual as well as from her mother; her obsessive rationality that divorces her pallid emotional response from her objective analysis of it. The patient's dream (and her inability to read it), Khan observes, stages an incomplete development of the mother-daughter relationship (*PRIVACY* 208). From his patient's subsequent recollections of and reflections on her dream, Khan reasons that the mother projected her own frustrations about her unhappy marriage upon "fetishistic over-involvement with her daughter's body hygiene" (*PRIVACY* 208) In the course of her daughter's upbringing, the mother imposed a rigid standard of behavior that denied the child the expression of any distress, anger, and aggression that the mother felt so compellingly toward a husband who had been absent from the home for very long intervals and who died when the patient was quite young. As a result of this enforced withholding, Khan concludes, the patient grew to be a highly intelligent adult with tendencies toward the overly rational.

Her innate sensitivity was blunted by an intense and unnamable insufficiency in herself (*PRIVACY* 206). Although possessing the capacity to hear, sympathize with, and support depressed friends, she could not understand why (Khan's emphasis) they were depressed (*PRIVACY* 206-07). She had lost access, said Khan, to an inner emotional life that could complete her.

Thus, the repetitive dream is Khan's female patient's way of staging an identification with a father she barely knew. Although physically withholding herself from the male element that he embodies (i,e., the closed casket), she nonetheless sees herself, through her father, as severely confined. Her mother has fabricated a narrow sexual "box" for her and refuses to let her out. Further, the mother's unloving laceration and abrasion of the father/daughter's face, along with the substitution of apples for the agency of sight (quite literally, the mother seems to have made the daughter the apple of her father's eye), prevents the child from perceiving self in her mother's gaze. With only defaced sensory equipment, the child can have no experience of self apart from "other", leaving that self emotionally dead and deeply buried.

Bizarre, to be sure. It's important to note that Khan's female patient isn't Linda, that there's no transferability of her dream to Linda, and nary the two shall meet. It's true that Linda suffered from disturbing dreams over a long period, though nothing quite as striking as the one Khan recreates.

But, as extreme as the Khan dream text is, there are some uncanny parallels with Linda's experience. The father in Khan's patient's dream presents like a dehumanized prop with only a vague history. Linda's dad, however, was quite different, while being just as central a figure, for Linda as well as her mom. Orien Clark was still a young man when he died (33), and he died a violent death as co-pilot on that ill-fated B-36. No question that he'd spent time away from the family in his reactivation during the Korean War. He'd left the Air Force in 1945 when he married

Traumatizing Linda

Dorothy in Florida, but, since his family was located in Yankton and Rapid City, South Dakota, they moved there and bought a tiny house thousands of miles from where Dorothy had grown up.

After working for a time in a TV and radio repair store in Rapid, Orien was called up at the onset of the Korean War and stationed at an air force base that would be renamed after the general who died beside him in the mountain-side crash in 1953. He and Dorothy had been married for eight years, apparently happily. I apologize for the pun, but it was true that Linda was the apple of her dad's eye. Though I know little of the specifics of their relationship, Linda told me often how he doted on her, how she idolized him, and how he walked her to her school directly across the street from their little house when he was available.

And then the fatal plane crash. At six, the loss of her father was numbing. And Dorothy, emotionally distraught, was barely able to attend Orien's interment at the National Cemetery in Spearfish before sweeping her two confused, bereft kids up and into the back seat of her '53 Pontiac and pointing it, with Linda recruited as navigator, toward Cupertino, California. Dorothy drove day and night over poor two-lane roads to one of Dorothy's cousins to do absolutely she knew not what. This was panic and emotional confusion, the truth of which was confirmed by Dorothy very shortly after piling her kids into the car and heading for East Boston. Crazy.

Linda barely talked about all this to me. She talked more about the few years—maybe three and a half—she lived, along with Dorothy and Richard, in a large three-decker filled with grandparents, sisters, uncles, aunts, and kids. But it didn't work. Dorothy wore out her welcome. Her depression, her torpor, her disinclination to work, her palming Linda off too often on the other kids and relatives in the house, left a mark on Linda, but it was nothing compared to the alienation she felt when Dorothy, with her sisters' assistance, bought the new little tract house in Braintree.

There, Dorothy immediately put Linda to work, making her as responsible as a ten year-old could be for doing all manner of household things that a chronic depression and lethargy prevented Dorothy from doing herself. On those occasions when Linda's work fell short of Dorothy's expectations, she received the full force of the hairbrush or whatever kitchen utensil was handy. Dorothy was a perverse combination of passive dying quail, heavy-lidded sleepiness in a state of undress unless she had no choice, helplessness along with what I and Linda had continued to see of her anger and cruelty.

So, I suppose, as a matter of clinical psychological correctness, neither Khan's nightmarish dream of mutilation experienced serially by his female patient nor my narration of Linda's roller-coaster ride through her sixth year after violently losing her dad and living through her mom's descent into the dissociated role of self-absorbed, tyrannical not-good-enough mother qualifies as classical trauma. There appears to have been no threat to Linda of her own physical death, or the fear of serious physical injury, as would be true of a person suffering from classic trauma of PTSD. Or the overwhelming belief that such a threat would visit Linda again and again (I'll revisit these questions in my final chapter).

I can't say categorically. I wasn't there, and, as was her way, Linda only divulged occasional hints of the anxiety that she must have felt at the sudden and permanent absence of a father she had loved and continued to venerate throughout her life. Not to mention the anxiety she had to feel traveling long distances through the night toward unknown destinations and living in crowded houses not her own.

Richard, on the other hand, appears to have largely escaped what Linda experienced. He was little more than a toddler, still entirely dependent on his mother who would summon whatever mothering energies and instincts to give to him what she could not give to Linda. Dorothy's unreserved love for Richard as her favorite would continue regardless of how nastily, as a teen, he would reject it.

Such a bundle of contradictions was Dorothy. Taking flight through the night in desperation to seek some security for herself and her kids, an act of apparent strength which was belied at every pass by inertia, an inability to self-motivate, seeking others' help and always believing, as I've noted earlier, she'd get it because of her belief in her physical attractiveness but never committing herself to another man, out of fear or venality, in order to protect the future financial prospects of the kids.

It's fair to say that Dorothy never finished anything. That was true of every painting she had attempted. A worn and frayed theatricalized still life that she would stage for anyone, including me, who entered her house.

After Linda and then Richard moved out and on, the house became a huddled fire-trap of unopened boxes of jewelry purchased in the middle of the night from the Home Shopping Network, teetering stacks and rows of containers filled with goods bought but never used with no room to move among them, rooms filled with broken or dilapidated furniture that Dorothy could barely make her way through, and a filthy kitchen whose refrigerator overflowed with rotten and spoiled containers of unidentifiable food.

When it became painfully obvious that the house was unsafe for Dorothy to live alone in and after she reluctantly surrendered her power of attorney to Linda, she and Karen flew back to Braintree and, in a long and dangerous week, sifted, garbage-bagged, salvaged, and dumpstered the house's contents and effected a house sale. By then, Dorothy, in full dementia, was moved into a nursing home a few miles from our Bloomington condo, all the while loudly protesting to anyone who would listen how she'd been kidnapped by Linda.

Dorothy's night flight years earlier had come full circle. The woman who had largely failed Linda as a mother while lifting Richard onto a pedestal had become her daughter's daughter—a daughter whose rage at her own mother's active indifference and passive-aggressive baiting of Linda's weaknesses was barely containable. Linda may have turned Khan's patient's dream upside down, with mother now squeezed in one closed box, the other box exposing her reason-less head. The motherly insufficiency and cruelty in Dorothy were unwanted gifts that kept on giving for Linda's entire life, even after full dementia had set in for Dorothy and her conflicted daughter found herself assuming the role of mother to her mother.

CHAPTER 13

Linda, We Hardly Knew Ye...

I don't mean the variation of the Irish traditional song title of this final chapter to be disrespectful, I assure you. If anything, my utter respect for Linda--the courage that she showed under so much pressure, how she managed to stumble, like Hans Castorp at the end of *Magic Mountain*, across the barb-wired and booby-trapped minefield of a mental battlefield that I'm still traversing so lovingly, and her strength against her own adversaries that would finally break--remains intact. Besides, it's true that, over sixty-one years and through all the cruel changes that can occur to people over time, we knew each other backwards and forwards, inside and out, good and bad.

But, in the period after her forced separation from Augsburg until the bitter end, I came to understand how little I could know of her. I used to joke with my students that we're all crazy, if just a little bit and only occasionally; after all, whether we were living in Hamlet's world, Yossarian's, or our own, we'd be crazy not to be crazy. And we'd be crazy to ever think that we could ever get to a point of fully knowing anyone. We are doomed to be isolates, aliens to one another.

After 1999, I felt Linda slipping away from me and from herself. She was retreating into a silence that would break only rarely by brilliant spots of joy—the birth of Karen's two children, Ezra and Lee; the long-awaited marriage of Chris to Geana and the birth of little Ronin who, tragically, because of having been born with the rare Cockayne Syndrome, would always be tiny and not have a full life's race to run.

In his book on trauma[8], entitled *The Body Keeps the Score: Brain, Mind, and Body in the Healing of Trauma*, Bessel van der Kolk cuts to the quick of Linda's mind and body shutdown. He states straight away that "trauma, by definition, is unbearable and intolerable…It takes tremendous energy to keep functioning while carrying the memory of terror and the shame of utter weakness and vulnerability" (*SCORE* 1). While van der Kolk makes clear that he is working with a "classical" definition of trauma focused upon the changes that have been wrought on survivors of war who carry home memories of horrific things they've seen and done as well as those who have survived the brutality of sexual depredation as children and adults, the symptomology of PTSD and sexual victims in case studies that he discusses bears striking similarities to Linda's predicament.

Before connecting some of the dots of that symptomology to Linda, I'll repeat what I've already said about what I cannot know for certain about what was happening inside her in her slide into depression and anxiety toward early dementia. Linda didn't/wouldn't talk. No sharing, ever, of what she was feeling or thinking. The world we shared grew ever quieter with my attempts to get her to tell me how she was doing, what she was thinking, who we might arrange to talk to her. Van der Kolk's book is filled with stories of veterans and victims who similarly couldn't talk about their memories, acted out ragefully the horror of the past that had become their perpetual present, and then, through talk therapy and other psychoanalytic strategies, had found ways to talk directly about it that gave them peace.

---

[8] See Bessel Van der Kolk's *The Body Keeps the Score: Brain, Mind, and Body in the Healing of Trauma* (New York: Penguin Random House, 2015). All future references to Van der Kolk's book will occur parenthetically as: *SCORE* #.

Because Linda wouldn't talk, I failed to understand, beyond her frustration and pain at the ways her body was failing her and the increasing lapses in her short-term memory, what was happening to her. When van der Kolk talks about trauma victims as "feeling dead inside" (*SCORE* 8), I could intuit this in Linda from her physical inertia and apathy. The evidence he presents of his patients expressing a lack of purpose or direction, a general "numbness," I could see in Linda and hear in her toneless lack of affect. "Imagination is absolutely critical to the quality of our lives," says van der Kolk (*SCORE* 11), and it was true of Linda in so many ways until she began, some ten years after she stopped working, to shed all her creative activities and sometimes even refuse to be among others her age who were doing them. I didn't need to be told that "alternate bouts of rage and periods of complete shutdown" (*SCORE* 20) were hallmarks of the trauma victim because I could see them in Linda,

If I could move van der Kolk's discussion of trauma out of and away from the actual battlefield, I would argue that what he says about trauma "result[ing] in a fundamental reorganization of the way mind and brain manage perceptions" (*SCORE* 24) describes Linda's unarticulated fixation on memories on her own internal battlefield. Do I believe that Linda, though unable or unwilling to express it, was suffering from dissociation and depersonalization, a "splitting off from the self" (*SCORE* 71)? Absolutely. As van der Kolk put it, she was in the survival mode of "making herself disappear" (*SCORE* 72-73). Whereas most of our everyday energies are spent "connecting with others" (81), Linda was bent on doing the opposite—damming up, shutting herself off, avoiding people she knew but wished not to see.

Dr. van der Kolk may or may not have wanted to include Linda among those whose experience of horrible war-time violence or sexual abuse caused them to replay the internal memories of those horrors unbidden, but my observation of her demonstrated all the signs of a body that had, indeed, kept the score of a cumulation of untreated traumas. From the beginning, there had been the low-level but sustained emotional abuse and neglect from a narcissistic mother to the point of barely being seen.

I can remember Linda having confided in me early in our relationship that, although she was a woman of great passion, she was frustrated by an inability to experience feeling in certain parts of her body, thus making intimacy difficult. As van der Kolk discovered, "many of my patients told me they could not feel whole areas of their body" (*SCORE* 97). The notion of one becoming separated from one's body Dr. van der Kolk connects back to Winnicott's work on the role of mothers (particularly, in Winnicott's phraseology, "good-enough mothers") in children's lives and "how our most intimate sense of self is created in our minute-to-minute exchanges with our caregivers" (*SCORE* 111)

Van der Kolk places great emphasis on attachment theory. It's common for a developing child to establish a strong "primary attachment bond" (*SCORE* 115) to at least one parent or caregiver. Doing so can provide stability for the child. Not having that strong attachment or having a caregiver who provides an "avoidant attachment" or "disorganized attachment" (*SCORE* 120-22) can send mixed messages to the child. Whether that incomplete or defective attachment be due to parents who are preoccupied by their own trauma (i.e., Dorothy's persisting mental paralysis over the death of her husband and emotional withdrawal), it's clear that Dorothy's lack of "attunement" to Linda's needs may have caused Linda to stop trying to make a positive attachment with Dorothy. That's where I found Linda at age sixteen—still seeking that attachment to Dorothy but always frustrated by failing to find it.

And then there is me. The loud knock by two police officers that brought Dorothy to the door at 1am, May 22nd, 1965, with an urgent request to speak with a Mrs. Dyer initiated not only the traumatic awareness that Linda's husband-in-stealth of one month was on the verge of death after a fatal car accident but also the entrance of Linda from that day forward into my own trauma. This would be our shared experience of PTSD— each of us from that moment became "a person suddenly and unexpectedly devastated by an atrocious event" (*SCORE* 177), never to be the same again.

But that huge trauma and the PTSD that Linda shared with me was worse for her. The heavy guilt I felt from the death of the young driver whom I had known only casually wouldn't let me go. I became obsessed with it, couldn't stop talking about it and the accident and the several reconstructive operations that went with it to anyone whom I could get to listen to me. And, of course, that meant Linda had to listen to the awful details of it as well as the rage, humiliation, and terror I felt considering the real possibility that I had lost myself and would never be a shadow of what I had been and might ever be. For every day of the ensuing nine months, I lay flat on my back alone in one of the upstairs bedrooms of my father's house encased in a Spiker cast from chest to the toe of my right foot maniacally reliving every minute of what I could remember and, when Linda returned home from work or her classes to care for me, I'd do it all over again for her.

If anyone needed a therapist, I did, but I wouldn't get one until I finally reached out to a small Bengali psychologist with an equally small practice in Mankato. I'd been having trouble doing my teaching job; I'd developed a large and heavy chip on my shoulder from the defenses I'd erected over some eighteen years as well as a rising number of jarring panic attacks. However, with the help of hypnosis, this kindly little gentleman succeeded in bringing my racing mind to a state of rest, and I was able to go forward with an open, confident, and peaceful self in my teaching and writing.

But it was 1983 by then. I had effectively drawn Linda into my trauma. Good for me that I'd found a means for finding my way out of the flashbacks and rage, but Linda was still carrying the burden of what I'd dumped on her. The fact that she never grew impatient with me or failed to empathize still brings a blush of shame when those memories flood back. It would just be a few years before Linda would find and then lose her own therapist and then inch closer to experiencing her own traumatic horrors and humiliations.

The final third of *The Body Keeps the Score* is all about finding and implementing creative ways to heal. First, the person beset with trauma must be made to realize the need for help and, with the insistence of those who love her, reach out for it. Taking that first step can be, as it was for Linda, impossibly difficult given the welter of possibilities of whom to contact and whether to commit to reveal the landscape of one's internal horrors to another. For Linda, those difficulties were magnified by the fact of her body failing her more rapidly than her mind. Linda was beyond some of the suggestions that van der Kolk makes, such as yoga or learning self-leadership or engaging in an activity that Linda had once appreciated, theatre.

Healing, he asserts, "requires owning the self" (*SCORE* 205). I agree with him when he quotes an expert of self-leadership, Richard Schwartz:

> Beneath the surface of the protective parts of trauma survivors there exists an undamaged essence, a self that is confident, curious, and calm, a Self that has been sheltered from destruction by the various protectors that have emerged in their efforts to ensure survival. Once those protectors trust that it is safe to separate, the Self will spontaneously emerge, and the parts can be enlisted in the healing process (*SCORE* 288).

I'd seen that self occasionally poking through in Linda. Even as Linda descended into the nightmare of dementia, not knowing where her home was but thinking, as she peered through our second-floor picture window at the assisted living facility where we lived, that "home" lay beyond the tree line in the middle of the woods. But I could watch Linda through that same picture window sitting around a garden table on the terrace below next to the pretty water feature with her caregiver Heidi over a three-hour span attempting to sort out the complex family entanglements of a young black woman sitting with them who was also contributing temporarily to Linda's care. Brilliant.

It might well have been Linda's original caregiver—her

mother—who held the key to her vulnerability to those traumas that entrapped her so many years later and that left her defenseless against her slide into dementia and the complications from Alzheimer's that followed. Says van der Kolk:
> It is one thing to process memories of trauma, but it is an entirely different matter to confront the inner void—the holes in the soul that result from not having been wanted, not having been seen, and not having been allowed to speak the truth. If your parents' faces never lit up when they looked at you, it's hard to know what it feels like to be loved and cherished…If you grow up unwanted and ignored, it is a major challenge to develop a visceral sense of agency and self-worth. (*SCORE* 298)

Although I wasn't there with her in her painful childhood, I know enough of it and of the years of belittling and baiting that followed to realize how fragile a foundation Linda's self was constructed upon from the synchronicity with van der Kolk's observation that his patients "could not erase the devastating imprints of a mother who was too depressed to notice them" (*SCORE* 299).

Healing requires taking full custody of the self. The multiple humiliations that Linda experienced and retreated from internally pushed her into an alternating rageful and sorrowful state of inertia. There could be no recovery without therapeutic intercession. Lacking that, Linda's only path was downhill into darkness.

AFTERWORD

...Since I Don't Have You...
--The Skyliners

...And I never will again. That's a tough one to accept. But, as I sit writing this final set of reflections in the cabin facing Lake Superior and the North Shore that Linda and I built thirty years ago, I know one thing: having Linda back would be wonderful, but not ever as she was in those months before she died. I've still got all her albums and scrap books that I can peruse to see who she was to us through the years until she wasn't, and there's real solace in that.

Several questions remain. Have I fulfilled my mission, articulated at the beginning of this manuscript, of demonstrating how the several traumas that Linda suffered led directly to the dementia and Alzheimer's Disease that killed her? No. I'll have to wait for definitive evidence from the neurological community to determine whether my argument holds water. And, although progress continues to be made toward a clear understanding of the causes and possible cures of Alzheimer's, I suspect that I'll be long gone before the ultimate answers arrive.

But it's important to say that my pursuit of a connection between Linda's untreated cumulative traumas over most of her life and the disease that ultimately killed her hasn't occurred without constructing and then following an evidentiary trail. I must bow humbly to the fact that the greater part of my "evidence" is anecdotal. That's largely because Linda left me no clinical resources to substantiate my anecdotes and her story. Of course, there was the wonderful and gentle Dr. Fuhrman who dealt directly with Linda, submitted her to tests, and wrote detailed reports on the state of decline he had found in Linda's cognitive skills. But such a skilled and highly experienced neurologist may have underestimated how quickly Linda's dementia would progress before accelerating into Alzheimer's. Not to say that Dr. Fuhrman was incorrect in any of his observations or diagnosis; in fact, Linda was clearly well into dementia when he performed his tests on her first visit, but his observation a year and a half later when Linda's behaviors worried Karen and me sufficiently to seek an update seemed to underestimate where she was and would soon be.

And that's not his fault. What a pernicious and unpredictable disease hers has been. It certainly would have been useful to have had the evaluations of Linda's mental state by trained therapists at various points along the way. Even a set of observations shared with me from the one therapist Linda invested in—particularly if her diagnosis of Linda's deep depression was concerning enough for her to recommend to Linda another therapist for Linda to continue to engage with—would have provided a beginning point for deepening an understanding what Linda was trying to cope with. The whole family could have enthusiastically supported her in her struggles.

All of which begs the larger question of when there will be full acceptance for the treatment of mental health issues as a normal part of public health. We don't yet. The stigma of mental decline currently dogs two presidential candidates, and one of those candidates has a history of mocking and criminalizing the mental defects of others.

Without any scientific evidence to go on, I've focused on three truths about dementia. First, women are more likely than men to be afflicted by it. Secondly, there's a congenital connection—in families in which previous generations have suffered from dementia, members of the current generation are much more likely to fall victims to it. Thirdly, individuals who have been subject to severe multiple head traumas over time are likely dementia candidates (certainly professional football players and prize fighters have often fallen into this category).

I'm convinced that Linda's career of mental decline accords with these three truths. However, I've attempted to build a special exception for her inclusion into the third one. I know of only one actual physical head trauma that Linda suffered during our long relationship—that fall onto and impact with the brick floor in a Minneapolis restaurant several years before she died. But I've recorded in this book the incidence of so many serious and life-altering events throughout her life that, although they don't fit the classic definition of trauma as Bessel van der Kolk understands it, in their cumulative totality fit his definition just the same. So many of them were severe destabilizing shocks that, much like physical concussions, begged for extended treatment. But she never sought that treatment, even though it was repeatedly recommended to her by Karen and me. And those severe mental concussions multiplied without treatment, some of them like the big three of the '90s occurring so close on the heels of the previous ones, and another all-consuming trauma leaving many invisible scars—the car accident that occurred just short of a month after we were secretly married—that she shared in co-dependency with me for well over twenty years. Assemble those brutal shocks together along with the unresolved shock of the loss of her father and the negligent care of a not-good-enough mother, as Winnicott surely would have described Dorothy, and one can see over time the withering of Linda's private and creative self to the point of debilitating silence.

Is that where her dementia begins? I don't know. But I do know that, when all of Linda's defenses against her rage, depression, and anxiety were spent, dementia took over. What's more, her violent launch into Alzheimer's was beyond anything I could ever have imagined. She still retained enough of her cognitive abilities, three months into Alzheimer's and only two months before it killed her, to look me squarely in the face from her bed and call me a "smudge-pot." Long-term memory stuff. One had to have shared her understanding from her youth what smudge-pots were and how they were used to know what she meant—not a nasty epithet, but, instead, a humorous mocking of my clumsiness in changing her soiled bed linens.

My experience with Alzheimer's was limited to case studies about people wandering away from their homes, forgetting the names of their loved ones or no longer knowing who they were or where they lived, suffering hallucinations, and finally, unable to swallow and then suffocating to death. Linda experienced hallucinations and the deadly oxygen deprivation at the end, but I'd not known before I saw it the absolute threshing machine that Alzheimer's could be. It came fully upon her just after the end of daylight savings time and dealt her terror, excruciating pain, and unspeakable indignities without fully depriving her of some portion of her faculties still able to know her torture. Five months of unmitigated hell.

If I haven't proven my argument that Linda's dementia/Alzheimer's was at least hastened by her career of cumulative trauma, I hope that I've demonstrated to my readers that going it alone as a caregiver is a fool's game. Do not do what I've done, or, to put it another way, don't try this at home. Up to a certain point, there may be nothing more admirable than a husband committing to the home care of a wife, or vice versa. But being able to humbly recognize that point and to deliver that spouse into the hands of competent caregivers requires a suppression of ego. I was too stubborn to realize that or, if I ever did, narcissistically blew right by it. Because of that, I often did more harm than good.

For those of you who are now caring for a loved one or expect to soon, get help. Often, good competent help is difficult to find. And, when it's good, frequently expensive. It will take time to find people who are truly qualified to do the work. Maybe multiple agencies or individual contractors will have to be tried before you find the right fit. Lots of frustrating wheel-spinning. Realize that the people who do good work for you are most frequently dreadfully underpaid and, thus, hard to retain. Hope to strike the gold of hiring people who establish an empathetic relationship with your spouse but realize how rare a thing that is. Do what you do best for your spouse—interact, play, talk, laugh, love, listen, and be present. Leave much of the rest—especially the stuff that causes you to have to invade your spouse's private spaces or dignity—to professionals unless your spouse insists that you do it.

And don't let the cost of outside care be the reason you've committed to doing it all yourself. There may be resources in the community, financial or otherwise, that can help. And there's the blessing of hospice. As I've said earlier, the cost of elite assisted living and memory care facilities is preposterous. But one can't put a price on community and the kinds of planned activities these facilities can provide. I'm even aware of one that enables a person in an assisted living unit to be transferred several times each week for several hours to memory care to improve that person's remaining quality of life. Get on the waiting lists of the ones you've visited and your spouse likes quickly.

Take care of yourself—there's life after this for you (and me). There's sanity to preserve. Think about what you're trying to accomplish with your caregiving. When might caring for a spouse become unproductive or conducing to greater discomfort, not to mention the potentially dangerous by putting your spouse at risk of injury? When might it be time for fools to stop rushing in where angels have feared to tread?

The full care of another requires constant focus and the stamina of a trained athlete. I didn't possess either. Instead, I ignored my health, went too often without sleep, and refused all the warnings about removing myself regularly from the caregiving process. I should have been seeking a therapist of my own. More regardful self-care might have helped soften my grieving process and shortened it. Or not. Nonetheless, loving (not loathing) oneself is not narcissism; it's the thing, says Erasmus in *Praise of Folly* (published in 1511), that makes it truly possible to love another.

Bill Dyer
August 2024

ABOUT THE AUTHOR

Originally from Boston's south shore, William D. Dyer grew up in the small bedroom community of Braintree filled with lots of academic promise, a good heart, and no common sense. Enlisted to become his mother's primary caregiver at seventeen, he tried to squander that promise when her cancer killed her by spending it all in two very brief encounters with distinguished institutions of higher learning. But, with help of his dauntless teenage spouse, Dyer got back on track, got his B.A., M.A., and Ph.D. and plied a successful forty-two-year career in college teaching. They shared two great kids and fifty-seven-year marriage before she succumbed to the horrors of Alzheimer's. Dyer and his Siamese cats now split time between a condo in Minneapolis and the cabin on Lake Superior that Dyer and Linda built together.

www.ingramcontent.com/pod-product-compliance
Lightning Source LLC
Chambersburg PA
CBHW020247010526
44107CB00002B/133